Pain: an ~~ambulance~~ perspective

Pain:
an ambulance
perspective

Edited by
Tracy Nicholls
and
Lucas Hawkes-Frost

CLASS HEALTH

Printing history
First published 2012

10 9 8 7 6 5 4 3 2 1

The authors and publishers welcome feedback from the users of this book. Please contact the publishers.

Class Health, The Exchange, Express Park, Bristol Road, Bridgwater, Somerset TA6 4RR, UK
Telephone: +44 (0)20 7371 2119
Fax: +44 (0)20 7371 2878
www.class.co.uk

The information presented in this book is accurate and current to the best of the authors' knowledge. The authors and publisher, however, make no guarantee as to, and assume no responsibility for, the correctness, sufficiency or completeness of such information or recommendation. The reader is advised to consult a doctor regarding all aspects of individual health care. Any product mentioned in the book should be used in accordance with the manufacturer's prescribing information and ultimate responsibility rests with the prescribing doctor. The authors and editors have made their best endeavours to locate copyright holders to secure the permission to reproduce copyright material. If you hold the copyright please contact Class Health, so that we may make the appropriate acknowledgement as to source and copyright-holder.

A CIP catalogue record for this book is available from the British Library.

ISBN 978-185959-345-5
E-book 978-1-85959-349-3

Designed and typeset by Typematter, Basingstoke

Printed and bound in the UK by Butler Tanner and Dennis Ltd, Frome, Somerset

Contents

Acknowledgements and contributors

Pain: an ambulance perspective coordinated, developed and contributed to by:

Tracy Nicholls, PGC (TLHE), FHEA, MCPara, Clinical General Manager

Lucas Hawkes-Frost, MCPara, Clinical Operations Manager

Chapter contributors

Tim Hayes, BA (Hons) PGCE DipIMC RCS (Ed) Cert HE MCPara, Clinical Operations Manager

Andrea Charles, MCPara, End of Life Care Champion

Michael Collins, Paramedic Clinical Dignity Champion

Ashley Richardson, FdSc, DipIMC RCS (Ed), MCPara, Paramedic

Jacqueline Stevenson, Paramedic Pain Champion

Nicola Draper, BSc (Hons), MCPara, Paramedic

Erica Ley, BSc (Hons), Paramedic HART Team

Daimon Wheddon, Clinical Operations Manager

Suzanne Lillington, Paramedic Regional Dementia Lead

Mark Eardley, MA, MSc, BSc (Hons), DipIMC RCS (Ed), Dip HE. Emergency Care Practitioner; Honorary Clinical tutor in Pain Management, Faculty of Anaesthesia, Critical Care and Pain Medicine, University of Edinburgh; and member of the International Association for the Study of Pain.

With thanks to the members of the Pain Focus Group

Allan Sunderland, MCPara, Paramedic

Andy Paterson, Paramedic

Danielle Garnett, Student Ambulance Paramedic

Gideon Chilton, Clinical Operations Manager, Paramedic

Daren Branch, Duty Operations Manager, Specialist Paramedic

John Martin, BSc (Hons), PGC (TLHE), FHEA, MC Para, Consultant Paramedic

Liz Morris

Mika Chan

Foreword

Across healthcare provision, pain is the most frequent trigger for patients to make contact. Within the ambulance service we encounter this every shift with regular calls for chest pain, back pain, abdominal pain, child birth and traumatic injury.

Working within the ambulance service is a privileged position where individuals place their trust in us by sharing their symptoms and history. They look on the individual who has responded to their 999 call as someone who is going to be able to help them.

When we undertook engagement in relation to the quality of care we provided we discovered that pain management was an area in which we could improve. This guide has been developed through the enthusiasm of a group of front-line clinicians who want to see practice enhanced. It explores the complexity of pain in physical, emotional and cognitive contexts and how this can be managed.

I hope this guide will allow all of those who use it to understand more about this common clinical symptom.

We as clinicians should accept the patient's report of pain, and ensure we treat their condition with the highest standard of care and compassion through the interventions we provide, from reassurance to intravenous pain relief.

Let us continue to improve and deliver excellence in the management of pain.

John Martin
Consultant Paramedic

Message from the East of England Pain Focus Group

Traditionally, pain was considered merely a physical symptom of illness or injury, a simple stimulus-response mechanism. Though the historic role of the health professions has been to relieve pain and suffering, there has been little understanding of the complexity of pain and only limited ways to manage it. Recent research shows pain to be a distinct disorder, with physical, emotional, and cognitive components. This view of pain has broadened our understanding of pain and given us new ways to understand its characteristics.

Pain is one of the most commonly reported symptoms of patients being cared for in a prehospital setting. Traditionally, the Ambulance Service as an entity, the primary provider of out-of-hospital emergency care, has struggled with the complex and complicated nature of thorough identification, assessment and management of pain in the wide range of patients encountered in day-to-day operations. Indeed, until relatively recently, analgesia was limited to the realms of splinting, entonox and inadequately effective analgesic drugs such as Nalbuphine.

The Ambulance Service, and paramedic profession as a whole, in the UK is undergoing a time of great change. With new roles and new extended scopes of practice becoming more commonly utilised within NHS Ambulance Services, a wider understanding and more robust approach to educating professionals about the nature of pain and more importantly, how to assess and manage it is becoming increasingly necessary.

This book seeks to be a guide for operational staff at all levels to provoke discussion, to introduce themes and practices that may be new to some and ultimately to increase the awareness and confidence of staff when managing the large number of patients we encounter who are in pain.

Pain is a unique and very personal experience, the management of which requires a great deal of sensitivity, understanding and confidence on the part of both patient and carer. It is sincerely hoped that the introduction of this guide will serve to bolster the capability of our front line operations to provide high quality, high impact, efficient, effective, goal focused personal pain relief.

Message from Hayden Newton, Chief Executive, East of England Ambulance Service

Welcome to our pain management guide for staff.

Our staff are faced with the challenge of managing patients who are in pain every day; it's an integral part of what we do. Reducing this suffering and pain is often a prime element of the reason we are called to help in an emergency. We clearly have a moral and professional responsibility to manage a patient's pain, but pain management is also important for humanitarian reasons. Improving the clinical care of our patients through pain management may also prevent further deterioration, which in turn will allow better assessment and will open up more referral options.

Patient safety and clinical quality is at the heart of what we do, and successful pain management plays a big part in improving the service that our patients receive. This guide will help to support our clinicians in delivering a high standard of patient care, and will help ensure that every patient receives the most effective pain relief that can safely be delivered. By doing this, we continue to fulfil our vision to be the leader in emergency and urgent care in the East of England, providing an exceptional standard of care of which both we and our patients can be proud.

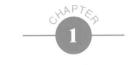

A road map to the guide

Lucas Hawkes-Frost

Summary

- Introduction
- Layout of the guide for clinicians

1.1 Introduction

In UK ambulance services, we see people in pain every day and pride ourselves in treating that pain, but without necessarily always truly grasping the underlying principles of pain or its devastating effects on the patients' lives. People who have chronic pain deal with daily life differently to those who suffer an acute illness or injury with its associated acute pain. Hence, it is important that we reflect our treatment regimens for all the patients we serve in our communities.

Working with our colleagues in the medical profession, we should provide a seamless analgesic armamentarium so that a patient who experiences any type of pain is provided with early relief from that pain. As the para-medic profession grows in maturity, we anticipate that our range of pain relief will grow to accommodate the many and complex needs of the patients within our communities, with the support of evidence-based research. This book is designed to encourage discussion and introduce themes amongst prehospital ambulance staff and keep pain management in the forefront of our assessment and treatment within the ever-evolving field of prehospital care.

This book seeks to provide clinical information that will underpin clinical decision making in a way that is comprehensive and accurate.

1.2 Layout of the guide

After this introductory chapter, the book begins by discussing the historical background to pain, covering the various theories that have arisen over time to explain the mechanisms of pain and its manifestations. Chapters 2 and 3 explore what pain is and describe some of the myths surrounding this experience. How it is assessed and measured is reviewed in Chapters 4 and 5, with commentary on the scales and tables currently in use.

The middle section of the book addresses pain in certain groups of patients: children, the elderly, those with dementia and those who are nearing the end of their lives. Assessment, ability to communicate and types of pain relief suitable for each group are covered in detail.

The final section of the book looks at the role of ambulance staff, the methods and drugs of pain relief that they have at their disposal, how roles interweave and how to deal with the patients themselves.

At the end of the book, Appendix 1 gives a table of drugs currently in use by most ambulance services for the relief of pain. This includes the scope of clinician currently able to administer those drugs. This is followed by a comprehensive Bibliography, much of which is cited in the text, but containing valuable resources for further reading.

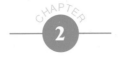
An introduction to pain

Lucas Hawkes-Frost and Tracy Nicholls

Summary

- Pain throughout history – William Morton's demonstration of ether inhalation.[185]

- Theories of pain – from Descartes to gate control theory: René Descartes *Treatise of Man*.[6] describing pain as a 'release of animal spirits'. Drs Melzack and Wall's discovery of the gate control theory of pain.[186]

- Experiences of pain – pain as a physical, emotional and bio-mechanical and cognitive experience affecting people in flexible ways.

- Definitions of pain – International Association for the Study of Pain defined pain as 'an unpleasant, subjective, sensory and emotional experience associated with actual or potential tissue damage or described in terms of such damage'.[8]

- Pain assessments – the patient is the only one who knows how the experience feels. McAfferey stated that it is 'not the responsibility of clients to prove they are in pain; it is the caregiver's responsibility to accept the client's report of pain'.[14]

- Treatment – can have physical, psychological, familial and social consequences if pain is left untreated or is poorly managed.

- Pain myths – fundamentalists cite the Bible as declaring that childbirth is a necessarily painful process. Brennan *et al*[4] put forward the theory that many people did not think that anyone would be able to help with their pain.

Summary continued

● Ethics and legalities – all paramedics must meet prescribed standards of clinical practice. Such standards are set to ensure safe and effective practice and to establish a code of accepted conduct, performance and ethics of registrants. The standards to which registrants work are broad, enabling them to make an informed professional judgement about each individual situation.

2.1 Pain throughout history

In the Museum of the Royal College of Anaesthetists, the following passage sums up the advent of the world of anaesthetics, the legacy of which we are benefitting from today. In September 1846 in Boston, Massachusetts, patient Eben Frost asked his dentist, William Thomas Green Morton, to mesmerise him in order to reduce the pain of surgery to remove an abscessed tooth. Morton offered instead to substitute the inhalation of sulphuric ether and performed the operation with great success.

Following this operation, Morton was invited to demonstrate his technique publicly at the Massachusetts General Hospital on 16 October 1846, administering ether to Gilbert Abbott. The Surgeon, John Collins Warren, wrote that, after breathing ether vapour from Morton's apparatus for about 3 minutes, Abbott sank into a 'deep state of insensibility' and then 'did not experience pain [...] although aware that the operation was proceeding'.[185]

Morton's role in this discovery is much debated by historians. The inebriating properties of ether had been suggested to him by his tutor Professor Charles Jackson. Morton's financial affairs were riddled with irregularities and the commercial possibilities of ether anaesthesia were not lost on him.

On 19 December 1846, in the presence of Francis Boott, an expatriate American physician who had received the news from Boston,

Massachusetts, the first ether anaesthetic in England was administered by dental surgeon James Robinson in Gower Street, only 2 months after the initial demonstration in the USA. Two days later Robert Liston operated on Frederick Churchill at University College Hospital and William Squire administered the anaesthesia – it was certainly quicker to roll out new clinical practices back then.

On hearing the news, Oliver Wendell Holmes, the celebrated writer and physician, triumphantly stated 'the deepest furrow in the knotted brow of agony has been smoothed forever.'[4] Yet 60 years later, in his preface to *The Doctor's Dilemma*, Shaw wrote: 'When doctors write or speak to the public about operations, they imply that chloroform has made surgery painless. People who have been operated upon know better.'[1]

Pain theories which predate even these examples can be attributed to French philosopher René Descartes, who in 1664, described the pain pathway in the *Treatise of Man* in the following extraordinary terms, 'Particles of heat activate a spot of skin attached by a fine thread to a valve in the brain where this activity opens the valve, allowing the animal spirits to flow from a cavity into the muscles causing them to flinch from the stimulus, turn the head and the eyes towards the affected body part, and move the hand and turn the body protectively.'[6]

Theories on pain and its management have now developed and the most comprehensive account of pain in all its forms with associated treatments is the *Textbook of Pain* by Wall and Melzack, the founders of the gate control theory.[13] Currently in its 5th edition, it is internationally recognised as the authoritative text on understanding pain and its management.

Our challenge is to translate a predominantly in-hospital treatment regime and adapt this to an out-of-hospital setting in emergency conditions, using evidence based medicine as our benchmark.

'Pain is whatever the sufferer says it is, existing whenever the sufferer says it does'. This concept can be challenging for many clinicians, whether working within community practice or in emergency care, such as the Ambulance Service.

Pain is a deeply personal experience and represents the most common trigger for patient contact with the medical profession. Pain informs us of dysfunction or injury in the systems or functions of the body and warns the sufferer that care and attention is required. Because pain is such a strong indicator of harm or disease and is a strong motivator for defensive or corrective action, it can safely be considered a prime warning and protection mechanism within the body. In addition, it is a symptom of significant clinical importance representing a patient's needs in a deeply unique and personal way.

In 1979, the International Association for the Study of Pain defined pain as 'an unpleasant, subjective, sensory and emotional experience associated with actual or potential tissue damage or described in terms of such damage.'[8, 74]

This definition gives rise to a number of questions about the actual nature of pain and its significance in the context of an individual sufferer. Pain, when considered as a delicate balance of physical sensation, bio-mechanical interaction, cognitive function and emotion is much more than simply a physical sensation caused by a physical stimulus. The experience of pain is deeply subjective, complex and personal, determined not only by biomechanical processes but by morbidity, co-morbidity, life experience, mental health, pharmacology and the overarching and centrally important consideration of how the individual patient views their own life and well-being.

In a variety of studies, pain assessment and scoring by clinical staff consistently underscores pain when compared with the scores that patients assigned themselves. This phenomenon exists throughout healthcare, where insecurity and reluctance to engage the patient in the process of assessing pain consistently under-manages the pain a person feels they are experiencing. As a profession, ambulance clinicians are generally confident and competent in assessing physical symptoms and baseline observations through a process of clerking that relies on objective quantitative measurements.

Measuring a patient's blood pressure is an objective observation that is not for interpretation and does not warrant debate. A patient's blood pressure is exactly as it shows on the sphygmomanometer. Pain cannot be objectively measured in the same way. Blood chemistry assessments are inflexible and not for debate; temperature is an inflexible measurement and is not for debate.

Pain is not so straightforward.

A patient's experience of pain is a flexible event that may change from one moment to the next, may change in nature, and may be affected by other illnesses, drugs, foods and living conditions in which the patient is found. Pain is a process that relies not only on the stimulus, but also the interpretation of the sensation. Pain cannot be measured in an objective way; pain cannot be quantified by simply looking at a patient and assigning a score. Pain is special and requires clinicians to hand over responsibility to, and be led by, the patient when arriving at an assessment of the pain that the patient says they are experiencing. This shift in control signifies a departure from clinical management that proves uncomfortable to a great many clinicians, irrespective of experience and level of clinical qualification.

How then will a clinician assess pain? If the assessment of pain is determined by the patient, then surely the patient must be placed as the leader in the assessment process. The patient is the only one who knows how the experience feels. In response to the concerns raised in emerging research around clinician-led pain scoring, the patient-led definition was developed by McCaffery (1979), who defined pain as 'whatever the experiencing person says it is, existing whenever he says it does.'[14]

In reply to the work of McCaffery, The American Pain Society felt it appropriate to apportion roles and responsibilities in assessment and management of pain, by adding that it is 'not the responsibility of clients to prove they are in pain; it is the caregiver's [sic] responsibility to accept the client's report of pain.'[14 158]

In terms of overall quality of living, pain is thought to affect the independence, mental health and overall social utility of patients more than any other health-related problem. This is consistently supported by findings from validated Quality of Life tools.[15]

7

Pain is strongly associated with interference in sleep cycles, mobility, cognitive function, independence, emotional stability, creative function, sexual function and self-actualisation. In addition to this, the theory of learned helplessness, developed by the positive psychologist Martin Seligman[16], suggests that patients suffering pain for even a relatively short period of time are at risk of descending to a point of feeling hopeless and helpless, their thoughts and feelings dominated by a sense of absent self-determination. Patients such as these are rendered virtually incapable of functioning through no more than repetition of negative stimulus.

To many clinicians, it will be of little surprise that, although pain is such a prevalent and pervasive symptom encountered in the world of clinical care, very little is known and understood about the processes and pathophysiologies of pain. Pain care, provided through the NHS, can be patchy, suffers to some extent with insufficient staff awareness and training, and remains a relatively low priority, especially in the realm of prehospital emergency care.

Reasons for deficiencies in pain management within the span of NHS clinical practice are widespread and include cultural, societal, religious, and political attitudes of both patients and the staff caring for them. In addition to this, the fundamental approach to the assessment, management and support of patients within the wider NHS often focuses on a predominantly *biomedical* model of disease, concentrating on pathophysiologies and symptom support rather than on a wider objective of improving quality of life. The biomedical model of medical care serves often to reinforce entrenched attitudes in some sectors that marginalise pain management as a priority when seeking to treat a patient.

As we enter the second decade of the 21st century, all evidence suggests a major gap between an increasingly sophisticated understanding of the mechanisms and pathophysiology of pain and the widespread inadequacy of its treatment, both in managing acute and chronic pain, throughout the NHS.

2.2 Consequences of undermanaging pain

Under-treatment of pain is the final consequence of healthcare systems not being familiar or confident with adequate methods of recognising, assessing and planning care for patients experiencing pain. Poor clinical practice results in a variety of adverse effects, both for the patient and for the clinician responsible for their care. In the context of a seriously ill patient, unrelieved pain is demonstrated to increase heart rate; it may have demonstrable effects on systemic vascular capacitance; and it may result in a marked increase in the levels of circulating catecholamine, placing patients at increased risk of myocardial ischemia, myocardial infarction, stroke, haemorrhage and clotting disorders, and other complications associated with their presenting condition. Inadequately managed acute pain commonly provokes pathophysiological neural alterations, which may include peripheral and central neuronal hypersensitizations that have been demonstrated to have the capacity to evolve into a collection of symptoms including chronic pain syndromes.

Chronic pain, closely associated with poorly managed episodes of acute pain, is linked strongly with a raft of physical, psychological, familial, and social consequences related to hyperexcitation of adaptive processes. In this regard, many adaptive responses to pain could be considered pathological entities in their own right.

From a physical point of view, such dysfunctional adaptive responses may include a sustained reduction in mobility, which later is responsible for muscle wasting and consequent loss of strength. Such effects have significant implications for the longer term well-being of a patient, significantly increasing the likelihood of falls and secondary illnesses associated with poor levels of independent mobility. In addition to this, patients often report disturbed sleep, increased susceptibility to illness, increased reported incidences of dependence on medication, and the development of codependent relationships with family members and caregivers.

Psychologically, the implications for mismanaging chronic pain are significant. In research commissioned by the World Health Organization (WHO)[135], it was revealed that individuals who live with chronic pain are four times more likely than those without pain to suffer from depression or anxiety, consistent with other statistics on chronic pain as a risk factor for both conditions. Persistent pain in patients with cancer interferes with the ability to sleep, eat, concentrate and interact with others.

2.3 Chronic pain and pain associated with oncological disease

A significant body of clinical evidence, mainly obtained from mature healthcare economies across the developed world, indicates that chronic pain represents a serious public health issue. In a number of studies, community-based surveys found that 15–25% of adults suffer from chronic pain at any given time, a figure that increases to 50% in those older than 65 years.[134, 135, 136, 137, 138]

Compounding the implication of the significant proportions of the population suffering chronic pain, is a prevailing fatalist outlook and feelings of helplessness suffered by those experiencing such pain. In a large survey of studies of pain, Brennan et al[4] observed that 18% of American patients who scored their pain as 'severe' or 'unbearable' had not visited any healthcare professional, thinking that nobody could relieve their suffering, further giving support to the Seligman theory of learned helplessness.[16]

These findings have significant implications for the ambulance and urgent care services operating within the United Kingdom. As services encountering many thousands of patients in an urgent or emergency context, ambulance clinicians are well placed to assess and manage patients not only on the condition they present with, which may indeed be pain, but also investigate the patient's wider health and social condition. With a robust approach to proactively assessing pain and involving patients in the process of quantifying that pain, ambulance personnel have a great deal of capacity to:

- Proactively identify unrecognised or undeclared pain
- Support patients in the assessment and investigation of the causes of that pain
- Effectively refer down appropriate care pathways to manage the patient's pain in the longer term.

The Brennan study[4] cites research of cancer patients' pain control that consistently suggests that up to half of patients in a community care setting report receiving insufficient pain management and around 30% do not receive appropriate pharmacological interventions for their pain at all.

The problems associated with insufficient pain management in cancer and end-of-life care are not restricted to the United Kingdom. In independent large studies of palliative cancer patients in France, the United States of America and China, the proportions of patients receiving insufficient analgesic support were 51%, 42% and 59%, respectively.[86, 87, 88, 89, 90, 91, 92, 93, 94, 95, 96, 97]

Revealed in an article published by the International Anesthesia Research Society, 80% of children dying of cancer in two Boston teaching hospitals experienced pain in the last month of life, according to a parental report. [58]

Less than 30% of parents questioned reported that management of their child's pain was successful and sufficient, and half of the parents described their children as having 'a great deal' or 'a lot' of suffering as the direct result of poorly controlled pain.

2.4 Basis for insufficient pain management

It is acknowledged that pain remains inadequately managed for a wide variety of reasons, including cultural (professional and societal), educational, legal and health system related reasons.

Evidence of human-kind's attempts at managing pain extends through thousands of years of human development. Throughout history, a pervasive narrative is present, spanning continents, cultures and technology describing the impact of pain on human life throughout the ages and the endeavours of those societies to understand and control pain in those suffering it.

Brennan et al point to evidence of the development of acupuncture by prehistoric humans in response to what was clearly a dramatic intrusion of pain on the societal structure and people at the time.[4] This surprisingly complex technological innovation, documented by recent studies of a Bronze Age cadaver, clearly displayed a network of tattoo work in the distribution of sciatic pain, likely associated with an arthritic condition.

Evidence exists across continents of early experiments with natural pain-relieving substances such as opium, belladonna, nightshade and

Mandragora, the effects of which may still be found committed to ancient records.

Brennan et al further point out that virtually all organised religions have taken a position on the problem of pain, to the extent that a great many religious and philosophical doctrines have 'saturated pain with meaning'.[4] Many examples exist of religious and societal influences on the management of pain. For example, fundamentalists cite the Bible as declaring that childbirth is a necessarily painful process.

Opposing both the church and powerful obstetricians, Queen Victoria requested that James Simpson administer chloroform analgesia for the delivery of her son, thus overcoming powerful negative attitudes that discouraged relief of the pain associated with childbirth.

2.5 Pain myths

All cultures and societies have clear and distinguishable outlooks and views on pain and on its treatment.

Despite a significant concentration of projects and campaigns by influential organisations and social and religious leaders, designed to improve pain management, cultural myths and those who promote them are well established and continue to spread throughout our multicultural society with ease. Throughout a great many cultures and professional outlooks represented within our own society, the belief that pain is an inevitable part of the human life is widespread and is accepted without challenge. Rather appropriately, the word 'patient' itself is derived from the Latin 'patiens', meaning 'one who suffers'.

Pain myths persevere and are shared by a great many health professionals and patients alike. These fallacies include the notions that pain is a necessary and natural symptom, representative of derangement in health and therefore a solid benchmark on which to base measurement of improvement and that pain is essential for diagnosis. A common healthcare myth that has been propagated, and may be to some extent an apocryphal example of behaviour experienced in the course of practice is, that the management of pain would 'mask the symptoms' and make subsequent diagnosis more difficult when the patient was assessed at the receiving health facility.

Myths such as these are further compounded by specific concerns about opioid and other forms of analgesia, which unfortunately abound within the realm of prehospital emergency care.

A concern of central importance, when considering improving the care of patients in pain, is ensuring that clinicians of all clinical skill level are competent and confident in accessing the full range of pharmacological pain relief options available to them. Principally, insecurity around the clinical use of morphine abounds among healthcare professionals, especially when using this powerful analgesic drug on a range of patients including those with polypharmacy, the elderly, patients with dementia and, most importantly, children.

Morphine emerged in the late 19th century both in China and in the West as an analgesic drug, derived from opium. Concerns among professionals appear to be based primarily around opioid addiction, rapid formation of tolerance and the risk of hyperalgesia. Opioid-induced *hyperalgesia or opioid-induced abnormal pain sensitivity* is a phenomenon associated with the long-term use of opioid drugs, including morphine, codeine, fentanyl, diamorphine and methadone.

When administered over time, and in some instances following single high doses, individuals receiving opioids have been reported in rare cases, to develop an increasing sensitivity to painful stimuli, even evolving a painful response to previously non-painful stimuli.[148, 149, 150, 151, 152, 153] Effectively, these patients become hypersensitive to stimuli that otherwise would not be associated with a pain response (allodynia). Some studies on animals have demonstrated this effect occurring after only a single high dose of opioids.[149]

Opiate tolerance and opioid-induced hyperalgesia both result in a similar need for dose modification, generally requiring a steadily increasing dose to achieve therapeutic effects. These phenomena are caused by two distinct mechanisms though, in a clinical setting, they can often prove difficult to distinguish from one another. Under long-term opioid treatment, tolerance (desensitisation of anti-nociceptive mechanisms), opioid-induced hyperalgesia (as described above), or a combination of both are common features of a patient's clinical presentation, requiring the clinician to balance the need for escalating doses to achieve effective pain relief, while maintaining an awareness of the potentially harmful side-effects of high-dose opiate therapies. Clinically, the identification of the development of, or indeed suspicion of, hyperalgesia is important. Patients receiving opioid drugs to relieve pain may paradoxically experience more pain as a result of treatment. This is a consideration that ambulance service clinicians need to be aware of, especially in the course of obtaining a functional enquiry of a patient's presenting pain and formulating a plan for managing the pain a patient reports in the course of assessment.

As Mao points out, an incremental increase in the dose of opioid is a proven means of overcoming tolerance; however, doing so to compensate for opioid-induced hyperalgesia may worsen the patient's condition by increasing sensitivity to pain while also escalating physical dependence.[149]

Although opioids are associated with a number of undesirable side effects, including hypotension, sedation and constipation, it is important to be mindful of the mild nature of these effects when opioids are utilised correctly. Many clinicians, including those within the ambulance service, have exaggerated concerns and attempt to mitigate such side effects. This is often achieved by shying away from the use of morphine and codeine, believing that opioid drugs are best reserved for only the most serious pain. **Morphine, like any other analgesic drug should be utilised as part of a step-wise approach to pain management, a so-called pain ladder (Figure 2.1).**

Many patients experiencing pain may believe that opioids can only be given parenterally. This belief often results in less analgesia being requested in an attempt to 'not make a fuss'. Clinicians, on the other hand, are often cited for withholding opioid/NSAID therapies, believing that analgesia may delay accurate initial diagnosis of an illness or condition.

Lastly, a pervasive attitude among many professionals maintains that at least some pain is inevitable, and that opioid therapies should be related to the perceived severity of the disease rather than the intensity of the pain being experienced by the sufferer. These beliefs, despite being manifestly incorrect, have a significant impact on the effectiveness of the clinical multi-disciplinary team in managing a patient's pain and have significant impacts on the quality of life a patient can expect to have when living in pain. Attitudes such as these recur in surveys of clinicians from a broad range of disciplines as well as in patients when asked about analgesia.[156, 157, 158, 159, 160, 161, 162]

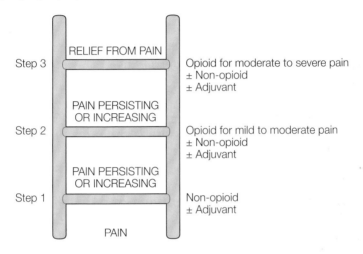

Figure 2.1 WHO pain relief ladder.

Opioid-phobia among health professionals is in many cases worsened by the phenomenon of 'opioid-ignorance'. In a series of surveys of health professionals responsible for morphine and with morphine administration, many clinical staff acknowledged that they had received insufficient training in, or exposure to, pain management as a stand-alone concept.[157, 158, 159, 160, 161, 162]

Many clinical practice shortcomings in providing adequate pain relief to patients trace their genesis, it would seem, back to insufficient under-standing and education.

Brennan et al highlight that many patients and the families of such patients express concerns about the use of morphine and opioid drugs because of a perceived association between these drugs with being an invalid and of old age.[4] Ignorance of drug options among patients from lower socio-economic backgrounds as well as lower levels of education have been identified as risk factors for seeking insufficient support from the clinical establishment in managing pain. Such concerns appear to be cross-cultural: studies in Puerto Rico, Taiwan, and the United States found similar views about the use of opioid medication.[92, 93, 94]

Brennan further points out that within branches of western society, redemptive qualities continue to be attributed to pain, such as withholding – or indeed denying – anesthesia for the soldiers in battle on the basis of a 'masculine cult of toughness and callousness'.[4]

Dismissive attitudes continue to inform the practice of medical and allied health professionals, contributing to myths about neonates not feeling pain and about elderly patients, or those suffering with dementia, not deserving the same level of analgesic intervention as patients able to effectively communicate their pain.

2.6 Ethical and legal implications of pain relief

When viewed through the prism of experience, time and technology, it seems unimaginable that pain management remains an area of clinical practice with such patchy application, clinical insecurity and low clinical priority. Indeed it is a relevant question to ask why it has seemingly taken so long for some to recognise the ethical and legal importance of pain relief as a fundamental right of all patients. The rationale for the delay in addressing this issue with the resources and commitment that is required is not easily packaged into a pithy statement suitable for this work. The issue of proactive and effective pain management is complex and contains many overlapping dimensions.

Throughout history, the medical and surgical establishments have prioritised the salvation of life over the management of specific aspects of a presenting medical or traumatic condition, especially where pain is concerned. This was especially the case in times when the technology and pharmacological capabilities of the clinical establishment were insufficient to adequately address pain. Until very recently, the level of understanding of the biomechanical and physiological process resulting in pain were patchy and insufficient to address pain and pain management as a pursuit, with a few notable exceptions, as the International Association of Anaesthetics points out, including the introduction of general anaesthesia.[3, 4, 5, 7, 9, 10]

The inception and development of the modern biomedical model of disease emphasised the management of a pathophysiology rather than the patient's quality of life. The distinction of symptom support from patient-centered support is an important one and perhaps represents the most compelling and important culture change that must yet occur within the realm of prehospital care if improved pain management is to be an achievable target for ambulance services throughout the UK.

With that in mind, perhaps our objective as a profession and as a publicly accountable agency should be to promote an objective, qualitative patient narrative rather than quantitative measurement of pain. Indeed, paramedics have, as registered health professionals, a number of responsibilities and obligations that apply as strongly to the management of pain as to any other area of clinical practice.

Although the Health Professions Council (HPC) has not produced guidance or policy specifically on pain management, all paramedics must meet prescribed standards of clinical practice. Such standards are set to ensure safe and effective practice and to establish a code of accepted conduct, performance and ethics of registrants. The standards to which registrants work are broad, enabling them to make an informed professional judgement about each individual situation.

Professionals must work within the limits of their knowledge, skills and experience. They must also act in the best interests of their service users at all times, making responsible and reasoned decisions, and seeking appropriate advice and support if necessary. Whilst the HPC – as a regulating body – has not produced guidance specifically on pain management there are general principles in our standards that would apply to these issues:

Standards of Conduct, Performance and Ethics: http://www.hpc-uk. org/aboutregistration/standards/standardsofconductperformanceandethics/

Standards of Proficiency for Paramedics: http://www.hpc-uk.org/publications/standards/index.asp?id=48

In terms of specific standards please note the following:

- Standard 1 of the Standards of Conduct, Performance and Ethics – 'You must act in the best interests of service users.'

- Standard 1a.1 of the Standards of Proficiency for Paramedics – 'be able to practise in accordance with current legislation governing the use of prescription-only medicines by paramedics.'

- Standard 3a.2 of the Standards of Proficiency for Paramedics – 'know how to select or modify approaches to meet the needs of patients, their relatives and carers, when presented in emergency and urgent situations.'

Ultimately, as a professional group, we have a responsibility to act in a way that is non-malfeasant, encourages autonomy and justice, and applies clinical care beneficently. As a network of professionals, ECAs, EMTs, Paramedics, Specialist and Advanced Paramedics (ECPs, CCPs), Doctors, responders, volunteers, we have a responsibility to meditate on the care we provide and take a stance of critical reflection. Entrenched attitudes to the management of pain and rationalisation of suboptimal practice persist, both within the healthcare establishment and in religious practice, as well as within the public domain. These beliefs include the notion that pain in childbirth is biblically preordained.

Health services within the UK are experiencing unprecedented demand from a public with ever-increasing and ever more optimistic expectations of the abilities of the medical establishment. As a professional, each clinician within a system as complex and wide reaching as the NHS has a responsibility to uphold the ethics of pain management. However, with the many challenges and demands on the service, ethics of pain management encounter barriers. Desensitisation and 'compassion fatigue' of health professionals surrounded by patients in pain may be widespread and must be addressed in order to better provide the necessary level of clinical care required of a profession.

The Hippocratic Oath states 'I will keep them from harm …' and its modern equivalent, the Declaration of Geneva, states 'the health of my patient will be my first consideration.'

The provision of pain relief as a matter of medical ethic is clearly established. The relief of pain is a classic example of the bioethical principle of beneficence. Central to the good actions of doctors is the relief of pain and suffering. As Post et al state, 'the ethical duty of beneficence is sufficient justification for providers to relieve the pain of those in their care'.[99] The principle of nonmaleficence prohibits the infliction of harm. Clearly, failing to reasonably treat a patient in pain causes harm; persistent inadequately treated pain has both physical and psychologic effects on the patient. Failing to act is a form of abandonment. As Somerville states 'many persons would rather be dead than unloved, abandoned and, too often, left in pain.'[4,113, 118]

2.7 Pain relief as an International Human Right

When the under-provision of pain relief is examined closely and compared to rights and responsibilities applied in principle at least to all humans, the right to live life free from pain insofar as possible appears increasingly credible as an insoluble human right.

As a concept, there is compelling support for such a move and there is some legal foundation for such a point of law. Interestingly, the International Association for the Study of Pain cites a number of existing United Nation (UN) statutes in support of the recognition of pain management as a fundamental human right as they state in their 'Declaration of Montreal'.[8] The articles referred to include:

- Appropriate assessment includes recording the results of assessment (e.g. pain as the '5th vital sign', can focus attention on unrelieved pain, triggering appropriate treatment interventions and adjustments). Appropriate treatment includes access to pain medications, including opioids and other essential medications for pain, and best-practice interdisciplinary and integrative non-pharmacological therapies, with access to professionals skilled in the safe and effective use of these medicines and treatments and supported by health policies, legal frameworks, and procedures to assure such access and prevent inappropriate use. Given the lack of adequately trained health professionals, this will require providing educational programmes regarding pain assessment and treatment in all of the healthcare professions and programmes within the community for community care workers delivering pain care. It also includes establishment of programmes in pain medicine for the education of specialist physicians in pain medicine and palliative medicine. Accreditation policies to assure appropriate standards of training and care should also be established.

- Failure to provide access to pain management violates the UN 1961 Single Convention on Narcotic Drugs declaring the medical use of narcotic drugs indispensable for the relief of pain and mandating adequate provision of narcotic drugs for medical use.

- The UN Universal Declaration of Human Rights (1948) (Article 5) states: 'No one shall be subjected to torture or to cruel, inhuman or degrading treatment...' Comment: Deliberately ignoring a patient's need for pain management or failing to call for specialised help if unable to achieve pain relief may represent a violation of Article 5.

- The UN Special Rapporteur on the Right to Health and the UN Special Rapporteur on the question of torture and other cruel, inhuman, and degrading treatment stated: 'The failure to ensure access to controlled medicines for the relief of pain and suffering threatens fundamental rights to health and to protection against cruel, inhuman and degrading treatment.'

In their treatise on pain, Brennan et al stress that international human rights are laid down in the foundation Covenants of the United Nations (UN).[4] The International Covenant on Economic, Social and Cultural Rights (ICESCR) articulates the right 'of everyone to the enjoyment of the highest attainable standard of physical and mental health' (Article 12). The Covenant obliges state parties to deliver on the rights it guarantees to the maximum of their available resources (Article 2). Although there is no mention of an express right to pain management, there is a strong argument that a right to pain management may be implied from the express right to health.

In summary, pain was traditionally considered merely a physical symptom of illness or injury, a simple stimulus-response mechanism. Though the historic role of health professionals has been to relieve pain and suffering, there has been little understanding of the complexity of pain and only limited ways to manage it. Recent research shows pain to be a distinct disorder, with physical, emotional, and cognitive components. This view of pain has broadened our understanding of pain and given us new ways to understand its characteristics.

So what is pain?

Lucas Hawkes-Frost, Tracy Nicholls and Erica Ley

Summary

- Pain modulation – pain is a sensation generated in the brain, after the receipt of sensory stimulus received through a number of neural pathways, which is modulated by two primary groups of naturally occurring and synthetic substances that work on the brain, CNS or peripheral tissues; namely, analgesics and anaesthetics.

- Inflammatory mediators – nociceptors are free nerve endings located throughout the body (except the brain). Their role is to respond to intense noxious stimuli. In inflammation, leukocytes collect at the injury site, producing redness and swelling.

- Gate control theory – the non-painful input closes the gate to the painful input, which results in the CNS not receiving painful stimuli.

- Pain mechanisms – natural pain suppression, somatic pain, visceral pain, psychomotor pain, referred pain, phantom pain and chronic pain.

- Sensitisation – previously inactive nociceptive neurones become active, increasing the painful stimulation being transmitted along peripheral afferent neurones to the CNS. In addition, tissue that has been affected by inflammatory changes for an extended length of time is thought to begin to release chemicals. These chemicals alter the physiological properties of nociceptive pain receptors, effectively causing them to become hypersensitive and initiating sensory activations seemingly spontaneously, and resulting in chronic pain for the sufferer.

3.1 Pain modulation

Pain is recognised as the most common reason for a patient to seek the assistance of the medical establishment. It is widely accepted that most, if not all, ailments of the body cause or have the capacity to cause pain in the sufferer.

Pain is a sensation generated in the brain, after the receipt of sensory stimulus received through a number of neural pathways, which is modulated by two primary groups of naturally occurring and synthetic substances that work on the brain, CNS or peripheral tissues; namely, analgesics and anaesthetics (Figure 3.1).

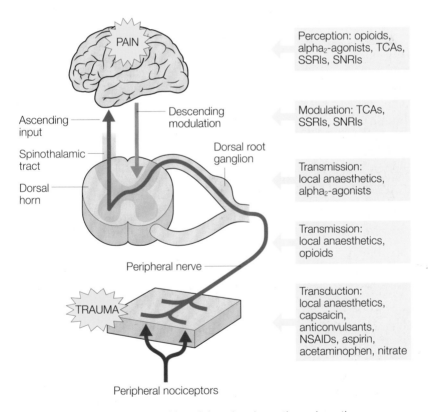

Figure 3.1 The effects of multimodal analgesia on the pain pathway.

3.2 **Inflammatory mediators**

As mentioned previously, nociceptors are free nerve endings located throughout the body (except the brain) (Figure 3.2). Their role is to respond to intense noxious stimuli. Thermal, mechanical and chemical stimuli form the categories of noxious substances.

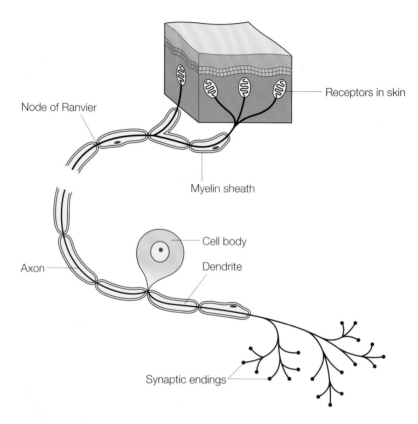

Receptors in skin

Node of Ranvier

Myelin sheath

Cell body

Axon

Dendrite

Synaptic endings

Figure 3.2 Diagram showing the sensory neuronal pathway.

Thermal stimuli are generally the consequence of a burn or scald. Mechanical stimuli may be the result of pressure such as tissue swelling, the presence of an abscess or indeed the formation of a neoplastic tumour. Chemical stimuli may also result from the activation of hyper-excitatory neurotransmitters, ischaemia and infection.

24

The cause of stimulation may be internal, such as a tumour, or external such as a burn. The category of stimulation is in fact inconsequential as following any type of noxious stimulation a host of chemical mediators are released in a process called transduction, resulting in the inflammation of affected tissues. The nerves responsible for conducting these impulses as well as their receptor types are detailed in Table 3.1.

Table 3.1 Types of nerves carrying impulses and their receptors

C fibres	A-delta fibres
Characteristics:	Characteristics:
1 Primary afferent fibres	1 Primary afferent fibres
2 Small diameter	2 Large diameter
3 Unmyelinated	3 Myelinated
4 Slow conducting	4 Fast conducting
Receptor type:	Receptor type:
1 Polymodal respond to more than one type of noxious stimuli:	1 High-threshold mechanoreceptors respond to mechanical stimuli over a certain intensity
2 Mechanical	
3 Thermal	
4 Chemical	
Pain quality:	Pain quality:
1 Diffuse	1 Well localised
2 Dull	2 Sharp
3 Burning	3 Stinging
4 Aching	4 Pricking
5 Referred to as 'slow' or 'second' pain	5 Referred to as 'fast' or 'first' pain

The transmission of pain occurs in three stages. From the site of injury, C fibre and A-delta fibres terminate in the dorsal horn of the spinal cord where a synaptic cleft bridges the terminal ends of the C fibre and A-delta fibres and the nociceptive dorsal horn neurons. In order for nervous impulses to cross the synaptic cleft, excitatory neurotransmitters are released including ATP, glutamate, calcitonin gene-related peptide, bradykinin, nitrous oxide and substance P. The impulse is then transmitted from the spinal cord to the brain stem and then through the connections between the thalamus, cortex and higher levels of the brain.

The end result of transmission of the nerve impulse is the perception of pain, which could be described as 'a multi-dimensional experience involving the reticular system, somatosensory cortex and the limbic system'.

Further chemical mediators are involved in the modulation of pain through multiple complex pathways occurring throughout the spinal cord known as the descending modulatory pain pathways (DMPP) leading to either an increase in transmission (excitatory) or a decrease in transmission (inhibitory). Inhibitory neurotransmitters include endogenous opioids, serotonin, norepinephirine, gamma-aminobutyric acid (GABA), neurotensin, acetylcholine and oxytocin, therefore producing analgesia.

However, it is only the transmission of pain which is inhibited. A pain impulse is still generated by the noxious stimuli that cause the release of inflammatory mediators that cause inflammation. We commonly understand inflammation to be a collection of leukocytes (white blood cells) which collect at the site of an injury causing increased permeability and movement of fluids and proteins into the tissues.

This response is characterised by pain, redness, heat and swelling, reflecting the four types of change in the local blood vessels. The objective of inflammation is to dispose of invading microbes, toxins or other foreign material at the site of an injury and to prevent their spread to other tissues.

Whenever body tissues are injured, the damaged cells release inflammatory chemicals in an attempt to combat the invasion and repair the cells to their functional state. This protective host response is part of the innate immune system. Whether the causative agent is infection or disruption in the integrity of the skin via an open wound, the processes that follow represent an orchestrated series of events in the quest for tissue repair.

An insult to the integrity of the tissues causes leakage of the cell contents into the extravascular space. This action exposes the sub-endothelial wall of blood vessels. This in turn activates the migration of platelets and the damaged cell membranes release thromboxanes and prostaglandins causing the blood vessel to spasm in an attempt to achieve haemostasis.

Activated platelets then release their granular contents into the blood plasma. These contents include serotonin, bradykinin, platelet activating factor, prostaglandins, prostacyclin, thromboxane A2 and histamine, which in turn activate additional platelets. This response lasts for approximately 5–10 minutes and is followed by an increase in vascular diameter leading to an increase in blood flow. This creates the signs of heat and redness.

In response to direct injury or on recognition of infection, mast cells residing within the affected tissues release their cellular contents, a process called mast cell degranulation; a process attributable to a substance called kinin. Kinin induces pain by directly stimulating nociceptors in skin, joints and muscle as well as sensitising them to heat and mechanical stimuli. The kinin system is another enzyme cascade relevant to inflammation. Kallikrein, derived from the inactive precursor prekallikrein, is activated by the action of Hageman factor. During inflammation, these substances leak out of the vessels due to increased membrane permeability and due to exposure to negatively charged surfaces the interaction of Hageman factor where prekallikrein is promoted to form kallikrein. High molecular weight kininogen (HMWK) comes into contact with kallikrein to form brady-kinin, a potent vasodilator whose pain stimulating actions are promoted by prostaglandins (Figure 3.3).

Preformed mediators (proteases, histamine and serotonin, heparin), newly formed lipid (fat) mediators (thromboxane, prostaglandin, leukotriene and platelet activating factor) and cytokines (eosinophil chemeotactic factor) are released from the mast cell into the extracellular environment. The bradykinin mediated depolaristation of nociceptors also induces a calcium influx into the cell causing both the release of neuropeptides such as substance P and the stimulation of arachidonic acid production. Arachidonic acid is produced through synthesis of phospholipid molecules from the damaged cell membranes by the enzymes phospholipase A2 and phospholipase C.

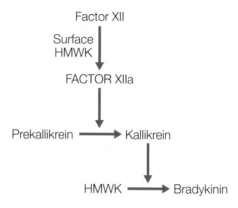

Figure 3.3 The Kinin enzyme cascade in inflammation.

Prostanoids (prostaglandins, thromboxanes, prostacyclin and hydroxy-acids) are then generated from arachidonic acid through the cyclo-oxygenase (COX) pathway and leukotrienes are formed through the lipoxygenase (LOX) pathway (see Figures 3.4 and 3.5).

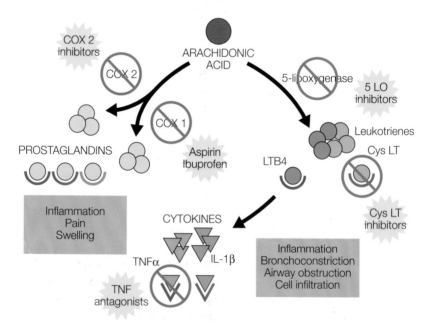

Figure 3.4 Production of inflammatory mediators from arachidonic acid.

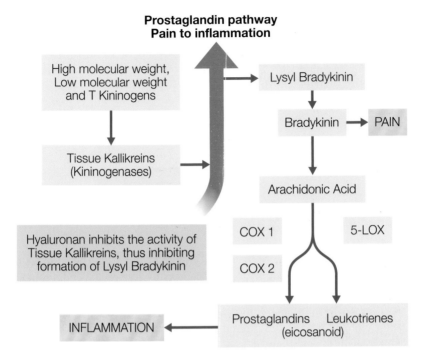

Prostaglandin pathway
Pain to inflammation

Figure 3.5 Prostaglandin pathway.

Currently there are three known COX isoenzymes: COX 1, COX 2 and COX 3. Prostaglandins are normally formed through the COX 1 pathway, yet during inflammation, formation is enhanced by the induction of a second pathway, COX 2. COX 3 is a variant of COX 1.

Prostaglandins do not directly effect nociceptors. However, due to their second messenger receptor coupling mechanism, prostaglandins inadvertently increase the activity of nociceptors. These second messenger systems also stimulate the release of substance P from sensory neurons. Substance P acts as a neurotransmitter and coexists with the excitatory neurotransmitter glutamate in primary afferent nerves (C fibres and A-Delta fibres) that respond to painful stimuli. It is thought to be involved in the perception of pain the in the brain. Substance P and its receptor, NK1, are widely distributed within the brain and are found in close association with serotonin and neurons containing noradrenaline in areas that regulate emotion.

29

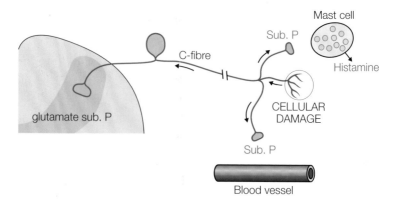

Figure 3.6 The axon reflex where some action potentials move peripherally.

Substance P is a potent vasodilator, the induction of which is dependent on nitric oxide release. However, NK1 receptors located on the endothelium are responsible for the vasodilation rather than those found centrally. The local release of substance P increases the local release of tissue necrosis factor alpha (TNFα) from injured nerves, which attracts monocytes and macrophages to the inflamed area. Substance P also stimulates the release of histamine by its action on mast cells. (Figure 3.6).

Histamine, released by a rise in cytosolic calcium, dilates post capillary venules and activates the endothelium (Figure 3.7). Small arteriole endothelial cells secrete nitric oxide, which causes relaxation of the underlying smooth muscle, and increases delivery of plasma and blood cells to the inflamed area.

During arteriolar vasodilation, a reduction in the velocity of blood also occurs, especially along the inner walls of the small blood vessels.

Endothelial cells lining the blood vessel wall become activated via the resident mast cell mediated release of the cytokines, TNFα and interleukin 1, which express adhesion molecules that promote the binding of neutrophils and monocytes. This combination of decreased velocity and adhesion molecules (leukotriene B4) allows the leukocytes to attach to the endothelium and following the production of chemokines, migrate into the tissues (extravasation), along the chemokine concentration gradient to the site of infection by way of a chemical signaling system (Figure 3.8).

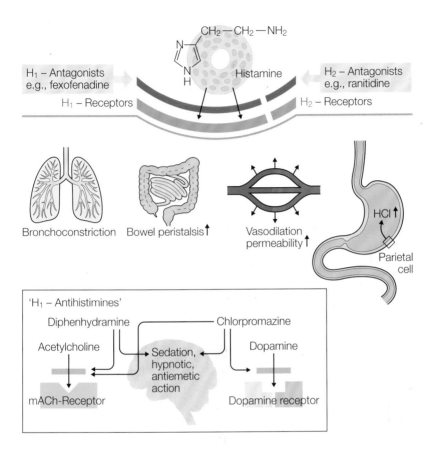

Figure 3.7 Summary of histamine actions on tissues such as bronchial smooth muscle, intestinal smooth muscle, bowel peristalsis and gastric mucosa.

Once in tissues, monocytes differentiate into macrophages. Macrophages and neutrophils ingest microbes and after binding with lysosomes, destroy them in intracellular vesicles via the substances reactive oxygen species (induced by leukotriene B4) and nitric oxide synthase; both of which are microbicidal. This process is called phagocytosis (Figure 3.9). Nitric oxide synthase causes an increased level of nitric oxide in the inflamed tissues, which contributes to swelling, hyperalgesia and pain. Macrophages also release TNFa which, in conjunction with prostanglandins and glutamate,

31

increase nerve cell communication resulting in a vicious cycle of inflammation. It is during hypoxic tissue reperfusion that reactive oxygen species are created in abundance increasing the production of cytokines, adhesion molecules and growth factors.

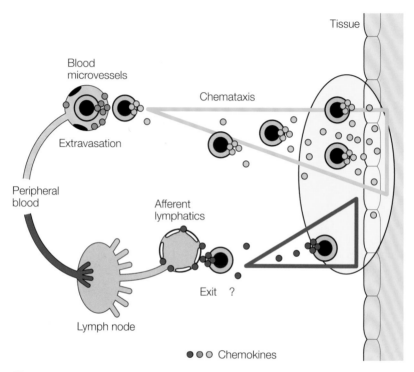

Figure 3.8 The role of chemokines in inflammation.

The result of increased vascular permeability causes fluid to leak out into the surrounding tissues causing swelling and, as a result, three enzyme cascades are initiated in addition to the kinin system mentioned earlier. The second system involves the adaptive immune system where immunoglobulins work to destroy bacteria. Following platelet activation (mentioned earlier) the coagulation cascade is initiated. Factor 7 is activated to factor 7a (by collagen) and the end product, fibrin is laid down in strands during a host-pathogen interaction as a method of trapping the microbe to limit the spread of infection. Thrombin is additionally involved in the activation of kinin and indirectly the fibrinolytic system.

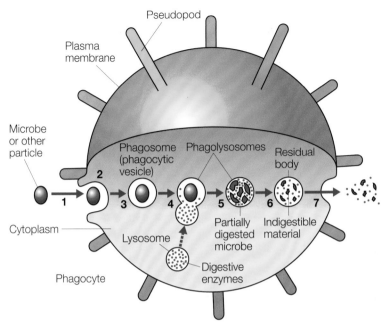

1 Chemotaxis and adherence of microbe to phagocyte

2 Ingestion of microbe by phagocyte

3 Formation of a phagosome

4 Fusion of the phagosome with a lysosome to form a phagolysosome

5 Digestion of ingested microbe by enzymes

6 Formation of residual body containing indigestible material

7 Discharge of waste materials

Figure 3.9 The phases of phagocytosis.

The complement system is a complex system of tissue and blood circulating proteins that are produced in the liver. In their inactive form, the complement proteins are numbered one to nine in the order in which they were discovered. Complement proteins act as a cascade resulting in an amplified net effect. The three different pathways of the complement system all activate C3. Once activated, C3 begins the cascade causing cleavage of C3 to C3a and C3b. C3b binds to the surface of pathogens causing a greater degree of phagocytosis by opsonisation. C5a functions as a chemoattractant resulting in the recruitment of inflammatory cells. C3a and C5a directly trigger the degranulation of mast cells as well as

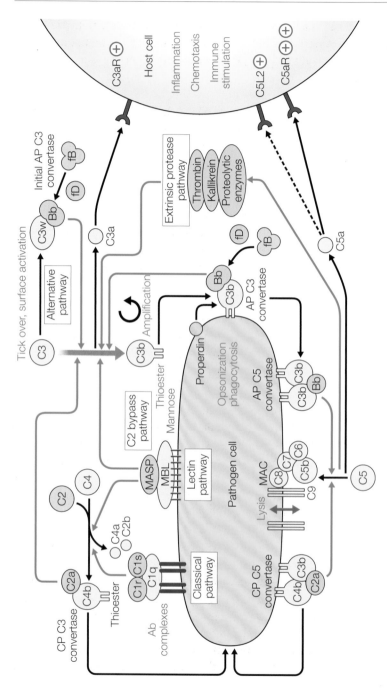

Figure 3.10 The complement cascade after activation by pathogens.

increasing vascular permeability and smooth muscle contraction. C5b initiates the membrane attack pathway resulting in membrane attack complex as an end stage of the complement system by osmotic lysis of the target cell (Figure 3.10).

There are vast mechanisms though which inflammatory chemicals produce and enhance pain. It is through the modulation and inhibition of these inflammatory mediators that pain and its perception can be minimised to improve the patient's experience and their prehospital journey.

In terms of functionality, the term analgesic refers generally to a drug or substance that relieves pain without loss of consciousness. In terms of modes of action, analgesic agents work centrally, that is, the drug depresses the central nervous function of the patient, for example morphine and benzodiazepines, and peripherally, that is, reduces the neural functionality at a local level, for example, paracetamol.

Anaesthetic agents, on the other hand, are characterised by the absence of or diminishment of perceived sensory stimulus, including loss of consciousness without loss of vital functions, for example cardiovascular function.

3.3 Opiate analgesia

In clinical practice, especially in the context of the ambulance service scope of practice, opiate drugs (naturally occurring or synthetic versions of drugs derived from opium) are considered to be the most effective clinically for producing temporary analgesia and relief from pain. These drugs, including codeine, diamorphine, morphine, fentanyl and pethidine, produce significant central nervous effects, reducing pain and offering significant euphoric and sedative effects.

Within standard scopes of practice, there currently exist no realistic alternatives to the group of drugs composing opiates. Several side effects resulting from opiate use include tolerance and drug dependence as well as the phenomenon known as hyperalgesia where, paradoxically, opiate-based pain management may in some cases lead to worsened pain.

Pharmacologically, opioid drugs modulate sensory information in spinal and central sites, thus preventing the receipt of pain information to the brain, as well as altering central functions such as thalamic sympathetic outflow, thus affecting blood pressure and other physiological parameters.

3.3.1 Endogenous opioids

Opioidergic neurotransmission occurs within the brain and spinal cord and is thought to have profound effects on the function of the central nervous system (CNS), including nociception (that is, pain stimulation), cardiovascular functions (blood pressure, cardiac preload, vascular capacitance), and thermoregulation (through the dense collection of morphine sensitive tissue in the hypothalamus), endocrine functions, respiration, as well as learning and memory. Opioids illicit marked effects on mood, and through the simulation of naturally occurring endorphins and encephalins, produce euphoria.

Broadly speaking, opiates exert their action on three primary classes of opioid receptors: μ-mu, δ-delta and κ-kappa. All three classes of opioid receptor are well represented throughout the brain and wider CNS, each of which represents the G-protein family of receptor targets. Similarly, three main classes of opioid peptides are believed to represent the vast majority of opiate interaction at receptor sites. These substances are the primary molecules responsible for interaction and activation with the above opiate receptors in the CNS and include: β-endorphins, encephalin and the dynorphins (Figure 3.11).

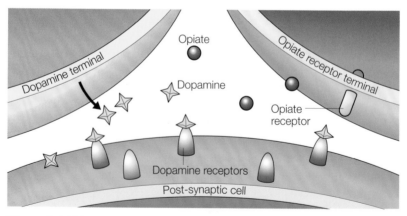

Figure 3.11 The activation of the μ-opioid receptors is associated with analgesia, sedation and euphoria.

Opioid substances influence nociceptive (pain) input through two main mechanisms:

1. Neurotransmitter release is blockaded through the inhibition of calcium ions (Ca^{2+}) influx into the presynaptic terminal of CNS neurones. The functional consequence of this is the prevention of action potential propagation along the neurone, thus effectively blockading a pain signal.

2. Potassium channels, also present within CNS neuronal cells, are chemically blocked in an 'open' position through a change in polarity, which effectively hyperpolarises neurons and inhibits the progress of action potentials within the CNS, effectively blocking the transmission of pain stimulus through the spinal cord.

The three primary classes of opioid receptor are distributed differently within the central and peripheral nervous system. This spread of opioid receptors suggests an explanation for functional differences in these receptors and their differing actions on a variety of tissues and physiological structures. The variation in receptor distribution also suggests a potential explanation for why many side effects occur following the administration of opiate therapies. An example of the biological rationale for these side-effects is mu (μ) receptors. These protein targets are widespread throughout the brain stem and chemoreceptive structures. Action on these receptors, closely linked with the respiratory centre, rapidly leads to an inhibition of neuronal function and therefore respiratory depression.

In terms of affecting nociceptive function, opioids influence afferent fibres containing opiate receptors, where natural and synthetic opioids act to retard an ability to transmit nociceptive (pain) information.

Systemically administered opioids, whether provided enterally or parenterally at analgesic doses, activate a series of spinal and supra-spinal mechanisms via μ, δ, and κ opioid receptors and intercept and interfere with pain signals.

Table 3.2 shows how the binding of an opioid to the different receptors is variable and the opioid's affinity to a subtype receptor has differing clinical features.

Table 3.2 The way in which opioids act with all receptors, including their subtypes (sigma and epsilon receptors)

Function	Receptor				
	μ	κ	σ	δ	ε
Analgesia cerebral	+	−	−	−	+
Spinal	+	+	+	−	−
Vigilance	−	↓	−	↑	−
Respiratory drive	↓	−	−	↑	−
Heart rate	↓			↑	
Cardiovascular tonus	−	↓	↓	−	−
Endocrine effects	+	−	+	−	−
Diuresis	↓	↑	−	−	−
Constipation	+	−	−	−	−

3.4 Gate control theory

Although the mechanisms of pain transmission and perception are to this day not entirely understood, it is commonly believed that within the CNS exists a biological circuit with which the brain is able to modify and interpret pain information being received from nociceptive (pain sensitive) neural pathways (see Figure 3.12).

The so-called 'gate control theory', as well as the 'ascending/descending pain transmission system' are two suggestions of such a circuit.

'Gate control' theory was first introduced by Drs Melzack and Wall in the middle of the 1960s.[186] Fundamentally, gate control proposes that non-painful input closes the gates to painful input, which results in prevention of the pain sensation from travelling to the CNS (i.e. non-noxious input (stimulation) suppresses pain). Gate theory remains the accepted rationale behind the pain-relieving effects of transcutaneous electrical nerve stimulation (TENS). In order to have a positive impact on pain, TENS units produce two distinct current frequencies, which fall below the pain threshold that can be tolerated by the patient.

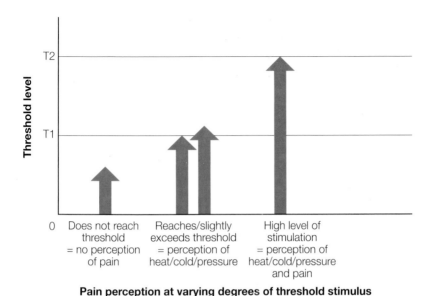

Pain perception at varying degrees of threshold stimulus

Figure 3.12a Pain perception at varying degrees of threshold stimulus.

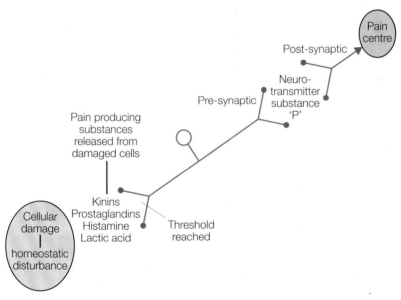

Figure 3.12b Diagram showing pathway from cellular damage to pain stimulus.

3.4.1 Ascending/descending pain transmission system.

The primary ascending pain fibres (the A δ and C fibres) reach the dorsal horn of the spinal cord from peripheral sites to innervate the nociceptor neurons. Cells then make synaptic connections and give rise to ascending spinothalamic tracts. At the spinal level, opiate receptors are located at the presynaptic ends of the nocineurons and at the interneural level layers IV to VII in the dorsal horn. Activation of opiate receptors at the interneuronal level produces hyperpolarisation of the neurons, which results in the inhibition of firing and the release of substance P, a neurotransmitter involved in pain transmission, thereby blocking pain transmission. The circuit that is contained within the grey matter then suppresses the descending pain, which inhibits incoming pain at the spinal cord level.

3.5 Pain mechanisms

Opioids interact with the opiate receptors at different CNS levels. Opiate receptors are the normal target sites for neurotransmitters and endogenous opiates such as the endorphins and encephalin. As a result of binding at the receptor, secondary changes occur which lead to a change in the electrical and physical conformation of neurons, thus modulating ascending pain information.

3.5.1 Somatic pain

Somatic pain is classified using two primary distinct sensation types; the first being cutaneous, superficial or peripheral pain and the second being a sensation referred to as deep pain. Cutaneous, superficial or peripheral pain is a type of pain that originates within the skin and muscles or indeed within the peripheral nerves themselves.

Generally speaking, somatic pain is composed of two main parts, the first being a so-called initial response and the second a later response. The two types of somatic pain, though most likely difficult to distinguish, are transmitted via two very distinct neural pathways. For example, a 'pricking pain' is transmitted to the CNS via the neospinothalamic tract, a relatively 'modern' area of human neurophysiology from an evolutionary point of view. On the other hand, pain described as 'burning or soreness', which arises through tissue damage, is transmitted to the CNS via the paleospinothalamic tract and archispinothalamic tract, two very primitive and basic areas of human neurophysiology.

Deep pain originates within joint receptors, tendons and deep tissues, known as fascia. Deep pain is often described by sufferers as dull, burning, or as an ache and is strongly associated with autonomic symptoms, such as sweating, nausea and even vagal influences such as transient hypotension. Somatic 'deep pain' is transmitted to the CNS mainly via the paleospinothalamic and archispinothalamic tracts. It is for this reason that deep pain is so strongly linked with autonomic symptoms, as a defence mechanism when tissue damage is sensed by the sufferer.

Somatic pain is usually the pain a patient feels when they experience sudden or unexpected damage to the skin or soft tissues. A response to this somatic stimulus is usually categorised as happening in three individual steps. These steps are:

1. Startle response: this complex series of reflexive actions is intended to quickly withdraw from the origin of the painful stimulus, through flexion reflex motion, possibly a postural adjustment to increase stability and facilitate movement away from the stimulus and a reflexive movement of the head and eyes to gain information and examine the damaged area of the body.

2. Strong autonomic response and arousal: in response to the information gathered and the change of position relative to the source of pain, the body releases adrenergic neurotransmitters, such as noradrenaline and adrenaline as well as hormones such as cortisol to raise autonomic readiness and prepare so-called 'fight or flight' mechanisms. By-products of these actions include peripheral vasoconstriction and other sympathetic effects.

3. Lastly, the body elicits a behavioural response, making vocal sounds, rubbing the affected area, as well as learning from the experience to be better prepared should such an injury occur in the future.

3.5.2 Visceral pain

Within the viscera (organs), tissues are richly supplied with nociceptive receptors which are sensitive to damage and irritation by stimulation such as pressure, chemical damage, ischaemia and physical trauma.

Generally, pain stimulation from the viscera is carried through a network of visceral afferent nerves; however the vast majority of sensations generated by nociceptive receptors in the viscera are not consciously recognised by the patient. Visceral pain tends to be diffuse in nature, be more difficult to apply description to and is strongly associated with autonomic symptoms such as bradycardia, hypotension, sweating and nausea. Visceral neural pathways are also responsible for generating sensations of hunger, thirst and make the patient aware of imbalances in electrolyte levels as well as respiratory or cardiovascular insufficiency – for example, chest pain associated with myocardial ischaemia.

Within the viscera, nerve endings are freely scattered throughout tissues, meaning that any stimulation which activates them has the capacity to cause visceral pain. Visceral stimuli are generally focused on spasms of the smooth muscle in a hollow structure, or distension of a ligament, such as a stone blocking the ureter or the gall ducts. Visceral pain may also be caused through chemical stimulation, for example, in the presence of gastrointestinal lesions and tumours, as well as thrombosis of an artery.

3.5.3 Neuropathic pain

Neuropathic pain is a devastating pain. Sufferers report persistent pain with little relief from conventional means of pain management. Neuropathic pain is thought to arise from a functional change in the central nervous system secondary to an injury affecting a peripheral nerve. Once damaged, a peripheral nerve may elicit continuous and sustained stimulation of nociceptors sending continuous pain signals along afferent nerves, which are processed as severe pain in the CNS.

Neuropathic pain occurs as a result of deranged activation of nociceptive neural pathways without stimulation of normal nociceptive pain receptors. Neural stimulation changes occur within the CNS secondary to the overwhelming afferent barrage and are thought to ultimately result in CNS neuronal hyperexcitment. Research has suggested that the phenomenon of 'sensitisation' of the nervous system following a peripheral neural injury is a factor in neuropathic pain. It is most commonly managed with NSAID group drugs to reduce afferent stimulation within peripheral neural tissues combined with long-term use of strong opioid drugs, such as fentanyl. When experienced as a result of certain illnesses causing neuropathy, such as in diabetes, AIDS and some cancers, pain relief is available in the forms of gabapentin and amitriptyline.

Neuropathic pain should not be confused with neurogenic pain, a term used to describe pain resulting from injury to a peripheral nerve but without necessarily implying any neuropathy.

3.5.4 Psychosomatic pain

The psychological effects of pain, both acute and chronic are well documented and well established within the realm of pain management. Psychological reactions to pain include a pantheon of responses such as anguish, anxiety, depression, nausea and muscular excitability through the body.

Psychological reactions to pain vary greatly between sufferers following comparable levels of pain stimulus. It is well established that the sensation of pain a person perceives can be strongly influenced by emotions, past experiences of pain and suggestions both of possible origins of pain or implications of such pain. The same stimulus can elicit different responses in different subjects under the same conditions.

3.5.5 Referred pain

Referred pain refers to a phenomenon whereby the sufferer experiences pain and discomfort at a location distant to the site of injury. Unusually, persons suffering referred pain report that pain experienced is not situated within the areas where it would most likely be expected; rather, it is localised to a distant site.

The exact mechanism for referred pain is not entirely clear. It is believed that the axons responsible for transmission of pain information from the viscera enter the spinal cord via the same route as transmissions carrying cutaneous pain sensations. Within the spinal cord, a convergence occurs of the information from both visceral and cutaneous neural pathways on the same nocineurons. The convergence of this information may explain the phenomenon of referred pain. Examples of the referral of pain in specific situations include pain associated with angina pectoris, or myocardial infarction. Many sufferers report that pain associated with these conditions is referred to the left chest, left shoulder and upper left arm.

- Cervical spine and occipitocervical junction disorders. (Dafny et al)[178]

Numerous studies both in and out of hospital have confirmed that acute pain is often inadequately managed. The reasons for this suggest:

- Lack of understanding of the nature and pathophysiology of pain
- Lack of understanding of the methods available to control pain
- Failure to assess the degree of pain for the individual patient.

3.7 What is pain?

Health professionals use different terms for different types of pain:

- Short-term pain is called Acute Pain. An example is a sprained ankle
- Long-term is called Persistent or Chronic Pain. Back trouble or arthritis are examples
- Pain that comes and goes is called Recurrent or Intermittent Pain, such as a toothache.

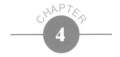

Assessing pain
– a practical guide

Jacqueline Stevenson

Summary

- Considerations during assessment – a guide to verbal and non-verbal cues when assessing a patient with pain.

Treatment of pain relies on taking a thorough history from your patient, but can also mean that the clinician needs to use some non-verbal cues to elicit the true nature and extent of their pain. As an ambulance service, we are called when a patient is in crisis or extremis. It is sometimes easy to forget how anxious people are when they have called and patients may feel very vulnerable about sharing so much detail with strangers, despite the situation.

Pain can make people feel humiliated as they feel a loss of control. It is important to consider that their attitude towards you may be affected by the fact that they are in pain. It can cause patients to become embarrassed and it may be displayed in frustration towards you during your assessment. As healthcare professionals it is crucial that we understand this and manage a patient's pain in order to alleviate these feelings and remove the pain.

Many things make assessing pain challenging; language, cognitive ability, culture, sensory loss or impairment, but a good clinician can use more subtle clues when assessing their patient and it is worth considering the following aspects when assessing a patient's pain.

4.1 Considerations during assessment

4.1.1 Listen to your patient

To really listen is one of the most helpful things you can do for a person in pain. Listening involves more than just hearing what is being said.

A good listener is able to read between the lines and interpret unspoken, non-verbal pain communications. To be a good listener you must focus your attention completely on the person you are communicating with, and listen to how they are saying it as well as what they are saying.

4.1.2 Be genuine

It can be unpleasant to listen to someone talk about their pain (imagine how it is for them). Do not ask someone how they are feeling unless you are really prepared to listen. However, it is better to really listen for just 5 minutes than to pretend – you do not have to have all the answers. People can tell if you are not really interested and it makes them feel like they are a burden.

4.1.3 Be aware your patient may not be completely honest

Many chronic pain sufferers are silent about their pain because they are so used to living with it and no longer see the point in telling anyone about it. Not expressing, or underreporting, pain are coping mechanisms that can be misleading. So when someone you suspect of being in pain says they feel fine, you can let them know that you are really interested, but you understand if they do not want to talk about it.

4.1.4 Be aware of your patient's body language

Chronic pain sufferers often underreport their pain, so look for a 'mis-match' between what is said and how they appear. Some tell-tale symptoms that usually indicate severe and inadequately controlled pain include sweating, irritability, sleep disturbance, restlessness, difficulty concentrating, decreased activity and suicidal thoughts.

Many chronic pain sufferers are so accustomed to these negative feelings they do not recognise their significance and so do not volunteer this information unless specifically asked.

4.1.5 Believe your patient when they say they are in pain

When pain sufferers complain about their pain, they are often not believed. There are many reasons for this including a myth that chronic pain sufferers exaggerate their pain in order to gain sympathy. In general, people do not go around pretending they are in pain to get sympathy – research[14] has shown that exaggerating or malingering are actually rare behaviours. Remember, 'Pain is whatever the experiencing person says it is, whenever the experiencing person says it does.'

4.1.6 Ask helpful questions of your patient

Helpful questions are specific or open-ended questions that let your patient know that you understand and are interested in the pain they are suffering. In addition to using the verbal numerical rating score in Chapter 5, other important areas to ask about include sleep, concentration, sweats and mood (look for depression, irritability).

It is amazing how rarely chronic pain sufferers are ever asked directly how satisfied they are with their treatment, and whether or not they think their pain is bearable. Being asked the right questions also gives the pain sufferer permission to talk about their pain.

4.1.7 Be aware of your own words

Thoughtless words such as 'you should see what other people put up with' or 'you don't look in pain' do nothing to help and only make your patient feel worse.

Just asking someone who is feeling at the end of their tether 'so how have you survived?' can evoke awareness of strengths and determination to continue.

4.1.8 Have compassion

Try and put aside your cares and preoccupations and listen with an open heart. Compassion is known to be one of the most healing human emotions.

4.1.9 Be honest about the limitations of your own knowledge

It is difficult to see a person in pain and not know how to help them.

Nobody likes to see someone suffer. It can be tempting to offer well-meaning advice such as 'you'll just have to learn to live with it', which, however well-intended, is not actually very helpful.

It is better to admit you do not know the answer rather than to say something which may unintentionally destroy hope.

4.1.10 Remember pain is not what you think it is

The concept of pain has undergone considerable revision in recent decades. Pain has gone from being thought of in purely physical terms to the realisation that it is made up of physical, psychological and neurological factors. However, although it is over 30 years since the *International Association for the Study of Pain*[7] officially declared that pain is both a mental and an emotional problem, many people still act as though pain can be understood simply as a sign of physical injury.

Pain is in part a psychological problem involving a range of emotions. The initial response to pain is fear, which is appropriate since pain represents a threat to identity and the ability to work, love and play. However, when pain persists, fear turns into anxiety and depression.

The effect of depression is for people in pain to show less emotion, and thus to not appear as though they are in pain. Pain is also very difficult to convey in language, making it even harder to understand what the pain sufferer is experiencing. So to understand a person in pain you have to remember that pain is a highly complex and individual thing.

The other thing to remember is that pain is different for everybody, depending on the personality and life history of the person experiencing it. Hence, it is difficult to imagine another person's pain.

CHAPTER
5

Scales, scores and tables: a comprehensive look at measuring pain

Nicola Draper

Summary

- Introduction – the assessment of pain should rely on the patient's self-report of their experience. Questions should then be asked that explore the characteristics of the patient's pain, including pain severity.

- Adults/older children – visual analogue scale, verbal numerical scale, verbal descriptor scale, McGill pain questionnaire, descriptor differential scale and brief pain inventory.

- Adults with mild cognitive impairment/middle-aged children – Iowa pain thermometer and colour analogue scale.

- Adults with severe cognitive impairment – Abbey pain scale, checklist of non-verbal indicators, Pain Assessment checklist for Seniors with Limited Ability to Communicate (PALSAC) and Pain Assessment in Advanced Dementia scale (PAINAD).

- Children – Wong Baker scale, Bieri scale, Oucher scale, Alder Hey Triage Pain Score Children's Hospital of Eastern Ontario Pain Scale (CHEOPS) and Face, Legs, Activity, Cry, Consolability scale (FLACC).

5.1 Introduction

Pain is a common presenting symptom for emergency patients. It is commonly difficult for clinicians to measure pain intensity due to the subjective nature of pain, which is only known to the sufferer. Although pain is a common presentation, it often remains undertreated[160].

Underestimation of pain has occurred when healthcare workers attempt to measure the severity of a person's pain experience. Therefore, the assessment of pain should rely on the patient's self-report of their experience. Questions should be asked that explore the characteristics of the patient's pain, including pain severity.

The assessment of pain is particularly challenging in the presence of severe cognitive impairment, communication difficulties or language and cultural barriers. Here, behavioural cues and changes to vital signs may be used to substantiate the patient's report.

Untreated pain can cause cardiovascular system changes due to sympathetic stimulation as a result of stress.[163] An increasing heart rate and blood pressure can be used in collaboration with the patient's self-report, although studies have suggested that there is a lack of correlation between pain severity and changes in vital signs prehospitally, therefore vital signs should not be used to estimate the severity of a person's pain.

In cases of pain in people with very severe cognitive/communication impairment, they may not be able to self-report pain even with full assistance. Therefore, clinicians may need to rely on behavioural responses alone, but these can be hard to interpret. [162]

There are many different methods for assessing an individual's interpretation of their intensity of pain, all of which have their own strengths and limitations. Many of these pain measurement tools have been rigorously tested and validated in the hospital environment; however, only a few are suitable for use prehospitally. Several facial actions characteristic of pain have been identified, including brow raising, brow lowering, cheek raising, eyelids tightening, nose wrinkling, lip corner pulling, chin raising and lip puckering.

Table 5.1 Shows observational changes associated with pain

Type	Description
Automatic changes	Pallor, sweating, tachypnoea, altered breathing patterns, tachycardia, hypertension
Facial expressions	Grimacing, wincing, frowning, rapid blinking, brow raising, brow lowering, cheek raising, eyelid tightening, nose wrinkling, lip corner pulling, chin raising, lip puckering
Body measurements	Altered gait, pacing, rocking, hand wringing, repetitive movements, increased tone, guarding, "bracing"
Verbalisations/ vocalisations	Sighing, grunting, groaning, moaning, screaming, calling out, aggressive/offensive speech
Interpersonal interactions	Aggression, withdrawal, resisting
Changes in activity patterns	Wandering, altered sleep, altered rest patterns
Mental status changes	Confusion, crying, distress, irritability

*Guarding = 'abnormal stiff, rigid or interrupted movement while, changing position'.

**Bracing = a stationary position in which a fully extended limb maintains and supports an abnormal weight distribution for at least three seconds.

5.2 Adults/older children with no cognitive impairment

5.2.1 Visual analogue scale

The visual analogue scale is commonly used for the rapid assessment of pain. The clinician uses a 100 mm line onto which the patient places a mark that is representative of the severity of their pain. The clinician then measures from the 'no pain' anchor to the intersection of the mark drawn by the patient and reports the pain intensity (Figure 5.1). This provides a pain rating score out of a possible 100. Reliability is reduced in people with visual impairment or cognitive impairment and has been shown to be less accurate in the elderly and young children. In fact, visual analogue scales are the least effective method for measuring the intensity of pain in older people.

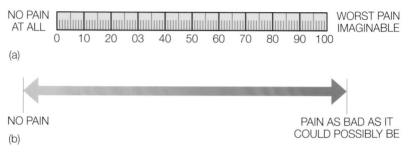

(a)

(b)

Figure 5.1 Visual analogue scale.

5.2.2 Verbal numerical rating scale

The verbal numerical rating scale is an easily applied measure. It requires the patient being asked to rate the intensity of their pain from an 11-point scale where 0 is considered 'no pain' up to 10 considered the 'worst possible pain'. This method has been validated in patients aged 13 and over. This has limitations in people with language and cultural barriers.

'What is your pain between 0 and 10, if 0 is no pain and 10 is the worst imaginable pain?'

5.2.3 Verbal descriptor scale

The verbal descriptor scale is based on the present pain index from the McGill Pain Questionnaire.[172] In this measure, a verbal descriptor scale ranges from 0 being 'none' to 5 being 'excruciating' pain, and the patients choose a descriptor of their pain as it is experienced 'right now'. It has been validated in both younger and older people.[160] There are varying versions of this, with between three and seven descriptors.

0 = No pain
1 = Mild pain
2 = Discomforting
3 = Distressing
4 = Intense
5 = Excruciating

5.2.4 McGill Pain Questionnaire

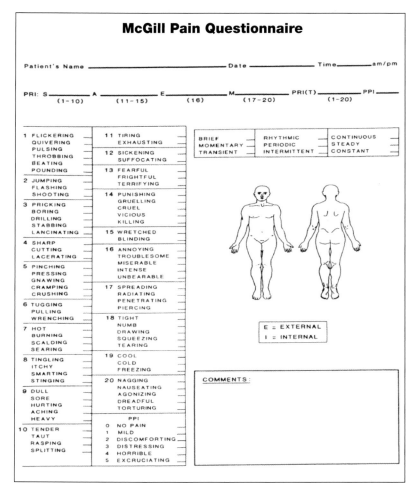

Figure 5.2 McGill Pain Questionnaire.

The McGill Pain Questionnaire (MPQ) is a standardised scale for the assessment of pain in cognitively intact adults. It assesses the sensory, affective and evaluative dimensions of pain. The score is calculated by giving a value to each of the descriptors based on the position of this descriptor within a word set and the sum of the values provides a pain rating index. The descriptors include sensory, affective, evaluative and miscellaneous. The MPQ is administered by reading a list of descriptors to a patient and asking them to choose a descriptor that best describes their pain at the moment (Figure 5.2).

The MPQ is reported to take 15 minutes to administer and score. Given this, it has limited application within the prehospital environment and questionable application within the emergency medicine setting.

5.2.5 Descriptor differential scale

The descriptor differential scale utilises two forms that measure separately the sensory intensity and pain affect (Figure 5.3). The sensations and pain affect are scored according to the amount that is present at that particular time by getting the patient to mark on the chart how strong the feeling is. This tool has been suggested to be too time consuming for the prehospital environment.

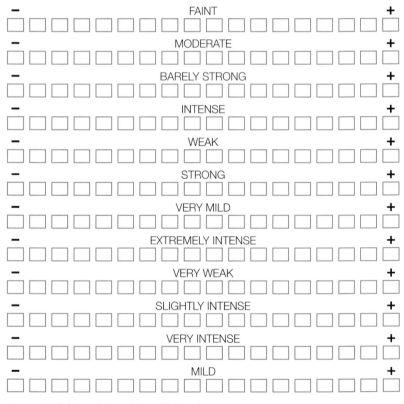

Figure 5.3 Descriptor differential scale.

5.2.6 The brief pain inventory

The brief pain inventory consists of 15-items that assess severity of pain, interference of daily activities due to pain, and impact of pain on mood and enjoyment of life (Figure 5.4). The pain interference scale uses an 11-point numerical scale; 0 being 'no interference' to 10 being 'interferes completely'. It aims to assess the interference as a result of pain in seven areas: general activity; mood; walking ability; normal work, including outside the home and housework; relations with other people; enjoyment of life; and sleep. It is well established at measuring chronic pain, but has not been evaluated for its use for acute pain and prehospital care. It is unlikely to be of benefit for the assessment of pain prehospitally.

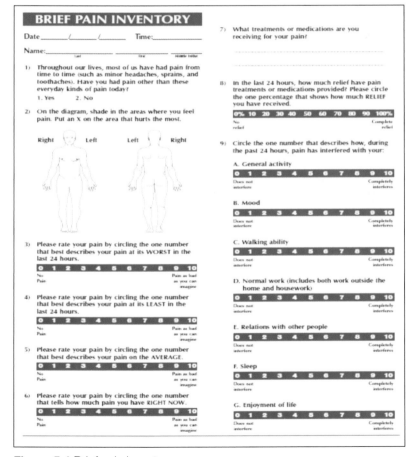

Figure 5.4 Brief pain inventory.

5.3 Adults with mild cognitive impairment/ middle-aged children

5.3.1 Iowa pain thermometer

This measure is an adaption of the verbal descriptor scale which aligns a thermometer alongside the options of words that represent varying levels of pain severity (Figure 5.5). Patients are shown the scale and asked to think that as temperature rises in a thermometer, pain also increases as you move to the top of the scale, and then point to the thermometer that shows how severe their pain is now. This scale has been validated in both older and younger persons, including persons with moderate to severe cognitive impairment. It has been shown to be the most preferred and easiest to understand tools for assessing pain in older persons.

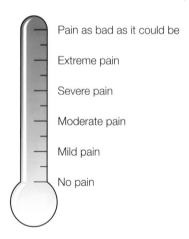

Point to the words that best show how bad or severe your pain is NOW

Pain as bad as it could be

Extreme pain

Severe pain

Moderate pain

Mild pain

No pain

Figure 5.5 Pain thermometer scale.

5.3.2 Colour analogue scale

This measurement tool is similar to the visual analogue scale and has the descriptors 'no pain' and 'most pain' at each end of the spectrum. The person slides the marker to the level of pain they are currently experiencing on the chart, the card is then turned over, which reveals numbers between 0 and 10 (Figure 5.6). The number that corresponds to where they have selected represents their pain score[160].

This tool is validated in children from age 5; however, it has been shown to be well understood in mid-stage Alzheimer's disease.

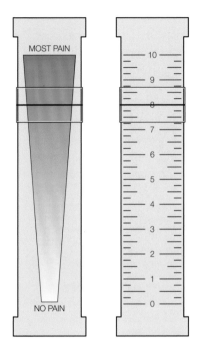

Figure 5.6 Colour analogue scale.

5.4 Adults with severe cognitive impairment

5.4.1 Abbey pain scale

This is used for the measurement of pain in people with dementia or other severe cognitive impairment that cannot verbalise. It is recommended that the assessment is completed when moving the patient; however, it forms part of an overall pain management plan, so it may not have a role prehospitally.

Each question is scored out of 3, then the total score calculated by the sum of each question, giving a total pain score between 0 and 18 (Figure 5.7). This can then be assessed against the score criteria which will give a pain level.

The Abbey Pain Scale

For measurement of pain in people with dementia who cannot verbalise.

How to use scale: While observing the resident, score questions 1 to 6.

Name of resident:...

Name and designation of person completing the scale:...

Date: .... Time: ....

Latest pain relief given was... at ....hrs.

Q1. Vocalisation
eg whimpering, groaning, crying   Q1 ☐
Absent 0   Mild 1   Moderate 2   Severe 3

Q2. Facial expression
eg looking tense, frowning, grimacing, looking frightened   Q2 ☐
Absent 0   Mild 1   Moderate 2   Severe 3

Q3. Change in body language
eg fidgeting, rocking, guarding part of body, withdrawn   Q3 ☐
Absent 0   Mild 1   Moderate 2   Severe 3

Q4. Behavioural change
eg increased confusion, refusing to eat, alteration in usual
patterns   Q4 ☐
Absent 0   Mild 1   Moderate 2   Severe 3

Q5. Physiological change
eg temperature, pulse or blood pressure outside normal
limits, perspiring, flushing of pallor   Q5 ☐
Absent 0   Mild 1   Moderate 2   Severe 3

Q6. Physical changes
eg skin tears, pressure areas, arthritis, contractures,
previous injuries   Q6 ☐
Absent 0   Mild 1   Moderate 2   Severe 3

Add scores for Q1 to Q6 and record here ➡ Total pain score ☐

Now tick the box that matches the Total Pain Score ➡	0–2 No pain	3–7 Mild	8–13 Moderate	14+ Severe

Finally, tick the box which matches the type of pain ➡	Chronic	Acute	Acute on chronic

Abbey J, De Bellis A, Piller N, Esterman A, Gilles L, Parker D, Lowcay B. The Abbey Pain Scale.
Funded by the JH & JD Gunn Medical Research Foundation 1998–2002.
(This document may be reproduced with this reference retained.)

Figure 5.7 The Abbey pain scale.

5.4.2 Checklist of non-verbal indicators

This is similar to the Abbey Pain Scale, and is indicated for use in adults who are unable to use other methods due to cognitive impairment. The measurement is conducted by scoring a '0' if the behaviour was not observed or a '1' if the behaviour was observed, giving a score out of 5 (Figure 5.8).

	With movement	At rest
Vocal complaints – nonverbal expression of pain demonstrated by moans, groans, grunts, cries, gasps, sighs		
Facial grimaces and winces – furrowed brow, narrowed eyes, tightened lips, dropped jaw, clenched teeth, distorted expression		
Bracing – clutching or holding onto siderails, bed, tray table, or affected area during movement		
Restlessness – constant or intermittent shifting of position, rocking, intermittent or constant hand motions, inability to keep still		
Rubbing – massaging affected area		
Vocal complaints – verbal expression of pain using words, e.g., 'ouch' or 'that hurts,' cursing during movement, or exclamations of protest, e.g. 'stop' or 'that's enough.'		
Total score		

Figure 5.8 Checklist of non-verbal indicators.

5.4.3 Pain assessment checklist for seniors with limited ability to communicate (PASLAC)

This measurement tool is for use in patients with dementia who are unable to communicate verbally. To use the tool, select the items on the form that were witnessed during the assessment. The sub-scales (facial expression, facial/body movement, social personality/mood, other) are then calculated by counting the number of items selected in each section. A total pain score is calculated as the sum of all four sub-scale totals (Figure 5.9).

Facial Expressions Present	Present
Grimacing	
Sad look	
Tighter face	
Dirty look	
Change in eyes (squinting, dull, bright, increased movement)	
Frowning	
Pain expression	
Grim face	
Clenching teeth	
Wincing	
Opening mouth	
Creasing forehead	
Screwing up nose	
Activity/Body Movement	
Fidgeting	
Pulling away	
Flinching	
Restless	
Pacing	
Wandering	
Trying to leave	
Refusing to leave	
Thrashing	

Activity/Body Movement	Present
Decreased activity	
Refusing medications	
Moving slow	
Impulsive behaviour (e.g., repetitive movements)	
Uncooperative/Resistant to care	
Guarding sore area	
Touching/holding sore area	
Limping	
Clenched fist	
Going into foetal position	
Stiff/rigid	
Social/Personality/Mood	
Physical aggression (e.g., pushing people and/or objects, scratching others, hitting others, striking, kicking)	
Verbal aggression	
Not wanting to be touched	
Not allowing people near	
Angry/Mad	
Throwing things	
Increased confusion	
Anxious	

Social/Personality	Present
Upset	
Agitated	
Cranky/Irritable	
Frustrated	
Other*	
Pale face	
Flushed, red face	
Teary eyed	
Sweating	
Shaking/trembling	
Cold & clammy	
Changes in sleep	
Decreased sleep or	
Increase sleep during day	
Changes in appetite	
Decreased appetite	
Increased appetite	
Screaming/Yelling	
Calling out (i.e. for help)	
Crying	
A specific sound or vocalisation for pain 'ow', 'ouch'	
Moaning and groaning	
Mumbling	
Grunting	

Figure 5.9 Pain assessment checklist for seniors with limited ability to communicate.

5.4.4 Pain assessment in advanced dementia scale (PAINAD)

The PAINAD Scale is a simple 5-item observational tool, developed and validated in 19 residents with advanced dementia.

To use this tool, the patient is observed, and then scored according to 5 criteria, with a maximum score of 2 for each section. This then gives a total score out of 10 for pain, with a higher score indicating more pain (Figure 5.10).

Items	0	1	2	Score
Breathing independent of vocalization	Normal	Occasional laboured breathing. Short period of hyperventilation.	Noisy laboured breathing. Long period of hyperventilation Cheyne-Stokes respirations.	
Negative	None	Occasional moan or groan. Low-level speech with a negative or disapproving quality.	Repeated troubled calling out. Loud moaning or groaning. Crying.	
Facial expression	Smiling or inexpressive	Sad, frightened. Frown.	Facial grimacing.	
Body language	Relaxed	Tense, distressed pacing. Fidgeting.	Rigid. Fists clenched. Knees pulled up. Pulling or pushing away. Striking out.	
Consolability	No need to console	Distracted or reassured by voice touch.	Unable to console, distract or reassure.	
			Total**	

Figure 5.10 Pain assessment in advanced dementia scale.

5.5 Children

5.5.1 Faces scale

There are two main face scales. Their use in the elderly is less effective than the verbal descriptor scale and the verbal numerical rating scale.

5.5.2 Wong and Baker faces pain scale

The Wong and Baker pain scale use six images of facial expressions, varying from a smiling face suggesting no pain to increasing intensities of pain (Figure 5.11). To use this method, the clinician should point to each face in turn describing the pain intensity associated to the face, the clinician should then ask the person to chose the face which best fits their pain and record the associated number. It is validated from 3 years of age. Wong and Baker faces pain scale is one of the approved pain assessment methods for children in the prehospital environment.

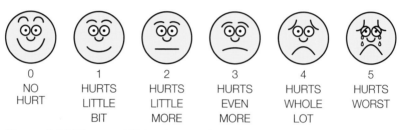

Figure 5.11 Wong and Baker faces pain scale.

5.5.3 Bieri scale

The Bieri scale uses seven pictures of facial expressions, although there are revised versions that show six faces assigned to numbers between 0 and 10 (Figure 5.11). The first face, which displays no pain as a neutral face, the other pictures display steadily increasing intensities of pain according to their facial expression. Its use is the same as the Wong and Baker, in that the child points to the face that best fits their own pain. This scale is recommended for use in children over age 5.

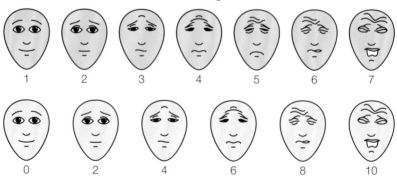

Figure 5.11 Bieri scale.

5.5.4 Oucher pain scale

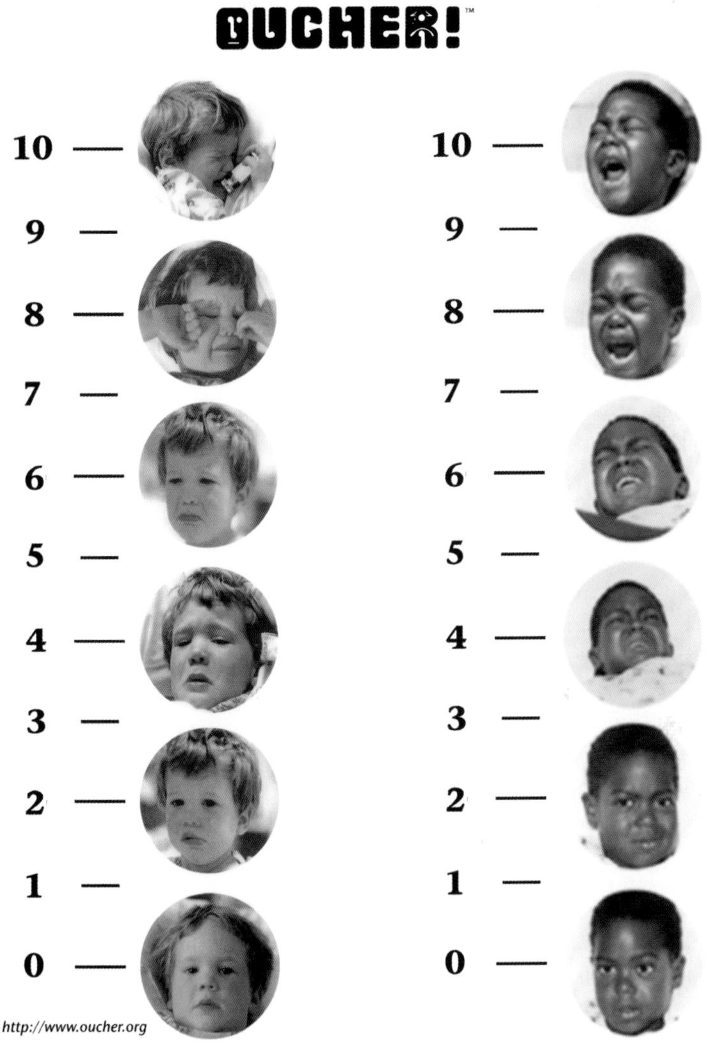

Figure 5.12 Oucher picture scale.

The Oucher scale is a pain scale used to measure pain in children. It combines pictures similar to those of the facial scales with a numerical scale. The picture scale (Figure 5.12) is for younger children and the number scale for older children. It has been validated in children aged 3–12 years of age, who need to be able to count to 100 and understand that 71 is larger than 49 to use the number scale, however the child should be asked which scale they wish to adopt. The scales come in different ethnicities (including Caucasian, African American, Hispanic, Asian boy, Asian girl, First Nations boy and First Nations girl).

To use the scale, the child should point to the picture which corresponds to their level of pain at present; this selection is then changed to a number score between 0 and 10. If the number score is used, then the child should point to the number which corresponds to their level of pain, that number is their pain score.

5.5.5 Alder Hey triage pain score

The Alder Hey triage pain score has been specifically designed for use in an emergency situation, and is completed by observing the patient. It is quick and easy to use, and can be completed with children aged 0–15 years. The child is observed and then scored between 0 and 2 for five sections, giving a total pain score out of 10 (Figure 5.13). It is recommended and can be used in the prehospital setting.

Response	Score 0	Score 1	Score 2
Cry or Voice	No cry/ complaint	Consolable, not talking, negative	Inconsolable, complaining of pain
Facial Expression	Normal	Short grimace <50% of the time	Long grimace >50% of the time
Posture	Normal	Touching/ rubbing/sparing	Defensive/tense
Movement	Normal	Reduced/ restless	Immobile/thrashing restless
Colour	Normal	Pale	Pale 'green'

Figure 5.13 Alder Hey triage pain score.

5.5.6 Children's Hospital of Eastern Ontario pain scale

This measurement tool was initially adopted for evaluating post operative pain in young children; however, it could be adopted for children in acute pain. It is intended for children aged 0–4. The score is calculated by the sum of the points for all six parameters, which will give a score between 4 and 13 (Figure 5.14).

Parameter	Finding	Points
cry	no cry	1
	moaning	2
	crying	2
	screaming	3
facial	smiling	0
	composed	1
	grimace	2
child verbal	positive	0
	none	1
	complaints other than pain	1
	pain complaints	2
	both pain and non-pain complaints	2
torso	neutral	1
	shifting	2
	tense	2
	shivering	2
	upright	2
	restrained	2
touch	not touching	1
	reach	2
	touch	2
	grab	2
	restrained	2
legs	neutral	1
	squirming kicking	2
	drawn up tensed	2
	standing	2
	restrained	2

Figure 5.14 Children's Hospital of Eastern Ontario pain scale.

5.5.7 Face, legs, activity, cry, consolability scale

The Face, Legs, Activity, Cry, Consolability scale (FLACC) scale has been designed as a behaviour pain assessment tool for use in non-verbal patients unable to provide reports of pain.

This scale is suitable for use in non-verbal children with cognitive impairment between the ages of 4 and 18; however, it is also suggested to be suitable for use in children under 3 without cognitive impairment.
The scale requires parental involvement and has only been validated to date in a hospital setting.

To use the scale, each section should be scored out of 2 by observing the patient and gaining parental history, these scores should be added together to give a total pain score out of 10 (Figure 5.15).

FLACC Scale (Face, legs, activity, cry, consolability)			
Face	**0** No particular expression or smile	**1** Occasional grimace or frown, withdrawn, disinterested	**2** Frequent to constant frown, clenched jaw, quivering chin
Legs	**0** Normal position or relaxed	**1** Uneasy, restless, tense	**2** Kicking, or legs drawn up
Activity	**0** Lying quietly, normal position	**1** Squirming, shifting back/forth	**2** Arched rigid or jerking
Cry	**0** No cry (awake or asleep)	**1** Moans or whimpers occasional complaint	**2** Crying steadily, screams or sobs frequent complaints
Consolability	**0** Content, relaxed	**1** Reassured by occasional touching, hugging, or 'talking to'. Distractible	**2** Difficult to console or comfort

Figure 5.15 FLACC scale.

Table 5.2 summarises the pain assessment tools that are available for use, according to age group and level of cognitive impairment. This list is by no means exhaustive.

Table 5. 2 Assessment tools

Children < 3 years	**Alder Hey Triage Pain Score** **Children's Hospital Eastern Ontario Pain Scale** **FLACC**
Children > 3 years, no cognitive impairment	**Faces Pain Scale (Wong and Baker, Birei)** **Oucher Pain Scale** **Alder Hey Triage Pain Score** **Iowa Pain Thermometer** **Colour Analogue Scale**
Older children, no cognitive impairment	**Verbal Descriptor Scale** **Faces Pain Scale (Wong and Baker, Bieri)** **Oucher Pain Scale** **Iowa Pain Thermometer** **Colour Analogue Scale**
Children with cognitive impairment	**FLACC** **Alder Hey Triage Pain Score**
Adults with no significant cognitive impairment	**Visual Analogue Scale** **Verbal Number Rating Scale** **Verbal Descriptor Scale** **McGill Pain Questionnaire** **Descriptor Differential Scale** **Brief Pain Inventory**
Adults with mild to moderate significant cognitive impairment	**Visual Analogue Scale** **Verbal Number Rating Scale** **Verbal Descriptor Scale**
Adults with moderate to severe significant cognitive impairment	**Iowa Pain Thermometer** **Coloured Visual Analogue Scale**
Adults with severe significant cognitive impairment	**Abbey Pain Scale** **PASLAC** **Checklist of Non-verbal Indicators** **PAINAD**
Elderly	**Pain Thermometer** **Verbal Descriptor Scale**

A variety of pain scoring mechanisms are recommended to encompass the wide variety of our patient population. Table 5.2 shows differing scoring and assessment tools that would enable a clinician to provide adequate opportunities for any patient to convey their experience and empower them to have an active part in their ongoing care and treatment.

Careful consideration should be used when deciding the most appropriate method, basing the decision on ease of use and practicality in a prehospital environment.

The most important factor is that a pain score is recorded and treatment given based on that pain score, not necessarily the method used.

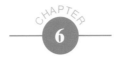

Children and pain

Lucas Hawkes-Frost

Summary

- Department of Health guidelines summary – children and young people have a right to appropriate prevention, assessment and control of their pain. There is still evidence that pain is inadequately dealt with for children.

- Pain relief in children – a clinician's anxiety and insecurities range from lack of exposure to children as patients to inadequate education or means of pain management.

- Assessment – assessment itself, however, is a challenging issue in children, especially in those children who are unable, either through age or development or indeed physical disability, to participate in explaining how they feel or understand the relationship between the treatment and the pain itself.

- Non-opiod analgesia – aspirin is not suitable for children. Paracetamol and opiods, along with entonox, are the only methods available in the prehospital setting.

6.1 Department of Health Guidelines

Children and young people have a right to appropriate prevention, assessment and control of their pain. There is still evidence that pain is inadequately dealt with for children, requiring better prevention, assessment and treatment. Thorough pain assessments are necessary and there are examples of some of these earlier in the guidance. Children who cannot express themselves should be given special attention. This includes babies, children with communication or learning difficulties, and those with altered consciousness or serious illness.

The treatment of pain using medicines requires appropriate choice of drug, dose, frequency, route and formulation. See Standards 7 and 10 (http://www.dh.gov.uk/en/Publicationsandstatistics/Publications/PublicationsPolicyAndGuidance/Browsable/DH_4867919) of the National Service Framework for Children Young People and Maternity Services: Children and Young People who are Ill.[180]

6.2 Pain relief in children

Managing pain and discomfort in children is cause for anxiety in a large number of prehospital clinician's minds. The reasons behind this anxiety and insecurity range from lack of exposure to children as patients, to inadequate education or means of pain management. As a result of this unease, pain is very often under-managed by ambulance staff, resulting in children remaining in pain significantly longer than is necessary.

Despite some commonly held beliefs, there is no evidence whatsoever to suggest that the pain a person experiences, even in utero, is any less severe and acute than an adult patient. Despite a developing nervous system, children experience pain just as their adult counterparts do. As a result of widespread belief in the idea that children experience pain differently, children tend to receive less analgesia than adults and drugs are generally discontinued sooner post injury or illness.

Further to this, children are often not provided with potent analgesic agents, such as opiates, because of concerns around side effects and addiction resulting from the use of these strong analgesic agents.

6.3 Assessment

As is the case with all pain management strategies, pain management in children depends largely on the ability of the health professional to identify and assess all factors contributing to pain in the paediatric patient, particularly the fear and anxiety experienced by the sufferer in conjunction with physical pain. In this context, explanation, patient involvement and participation of the patient and their parents if appropriate in the process of managing pain can be as useful in treatment as the analgesic itself.

Assessment itself, however, is a challenging issue in children, especially in those children who are unable, either through age or development or indeed physical disability, to participate in explaining how they feel or understand the relationship between the treatment and the pain itself.

In very young patients, observational pain assessment scales may be found to be useful, including observations of the face, legs, activity, cry and consolability (the FLACC scale), championed by the Great Ormond Street Hospital (see Chapter 5). Observational measures are of great benefit to the clinician; however, it is worth highlighting that the absence of outward signs of pain in children does not necessarily rule out the existence of pain. Features such as noting the position of the child, their sleeping patterns, feeding, pitch of cry, consolability, parental response and muscle tone all contribute to creating an impression and a cumulative pain score.

In children over the age of 4, pain assessment scales utilising colours, pictures of faces, expressions and even visual analogue scales may be useful in building an impression of the level of pain a child may or may not be suffering (see Chapter 5).

Crucially, the management of pain in children must, by its very nature, be a more active one than the process utilised in the assessment of pain in adults. Greater emphasis must be placed on the need for the clinician to anticipate pain and to therefore manage pain in a much more proactive way. Children must never be relied on to make the clinician aware of the pain they are suffering; rather the children should be placed in a position of central importance in describing their pain response secondary to a proactive pain management regime which makes use of the variety of pain relief tools at the disposal of the ambulance clinician.

It is preferable to utilise the 'pain ladder' approach as treating immediately with pharmacological methods can often be fraught, for both the child and the clinician. Where appropriate, try simple things to relieve the pain, which may also help with the psychological issues of trust with the child. If pharmacological treatment is required, again, start with simple analgesia and work up the pain ladder.

Preferred methods of drug delivery depend to a large extent on the specific drug selected, the nature and perceived severity of the pain the patient is experiencing and the desired timeline and acceptable side-effects. In children, it is preferable, where possible, to administer drugs enterally, thereby reducing the necessity for injection and venipuncture, causes of pain and anxiety in themselves. In the context of ambulance service care, the introduction of oral morphine has provided an additional means of analgesia in children, thereby avoiding administering any invasive procedures. Alternatively, administration of medications rectally is beneficial in many cases, owing to rapid absorption, relatively predictable action and lack of fear and anxiety associated with injections. Rectal drug administration is especially desirable where the patient is vomiting concurrently with their pain and unable to tolerate oral analgesics.

Parenterally administered analgesics have a number of practical benefits for the ambulance clinician, most obviously that the pharmacological action of the drug given is almost instantaneous, with the maximum analgesic effect being reached in 10–20 minutes. In addition to this, much more sensitive dosing of analgesic drugs can be achieved with parenteral administration. However, many drawbacks exist, including the pain and fear experienced by most children undergoing an injection, that should make the clinician consider whether it is necessary to provide IV analgesia, or whether alternative drugs or administration routes would be more appropriate. In children, intramuscular injections should be avoided as they may be very painful themselves, especially when administered in any volume greater than fractions of a millilitre.

Where intravenous drug administration is not avoidable, topical analgesic creams are available and in widespread use that when applied beneath an occlusive dressing, will provide anaesthesia of the skin for greater than an hour. These creams, including Tetracaine, reduce the unpleasant sensation and pain associated with IV cannulation and infiltration of local anaesthetic agents (within the specialist paramedic scope of practice). They also reduce stress and fear in the child by involving them in the process and giving a focus which is not directly the process of cannulation. Obviously, topical creams such as Tetracaine cannot be applied directly to a wound or mucous membrane; however, they do provide a painless area of skin through which to administer analgesia or provide venous access.

It is worth noting that many procedures and practices associated with analgesia can ironically be quite painful themselves.

In cases of significant limb trauma in children, it is worth noting that a number of BASICS and HEMS schemes operating within the prehospital arena offer regional anaesthesia, including regional nerve blocks. This procedure involves the infiltration of a strong anaesthetic agent around a regional nerve plexus. Drugs used in this procedure commonly include agents such as Bupivicaine, a strong anaesthetic drug that elicits a blockade on voltage gated sodium channels within neural tissue. Through the blockade of these channels, nerve impulses from nociceptive pain receptors are blocked, effectively anaesthetising an entire limb in isolation, without the complicated procedures associated with a general anaesthesia.

6.4 Non-opioid analgesia

Paracetamol is an effective and well-established analgesic and anti-pyrexial drug within the paramedic and EMT scope of practice, having significant effects on mild to moderate pain, especially secondary to inflammation. Paracetamol can be administered orally, rectally and via an intravenous route and has been demonstrated to be highly effective in managing pain from a wide range of pathophysiologies.

The MHRA has recently revised guidelines on the dosing of paracetamol, which can be found on their web site.[182]

6.4.1 Background

The current recommended doses consist of wide age bands with the option to receive 5 ml or 10 ml within each dose range. As a result, children who are light for their age and receive the maximum recommended dose will receive an amount per kg bodyweight that differs from older, heavier children taking the lower recommended dose within that age band. Consequently, lighter children may currently be receiving a higher dose than needed for an effective therapeutic result, if the parent or carer decides to use the larger dosing option.

To address this, the dosing for liquid paracetamol products for children has been revised to one that is based on narrower age bands with a single dosing option per band. Although dosing for children on mg/kg body-weight is standard practice in hospitals, this is not always practical for parents to manage at home. The new posology retains dosing by age bands and the familiar 2.5 ml and 5.0 ml increments.

The changes to paediatric paracetamol dosing have not altered the dose of paracetamol recommended for the treatment of post-vaccination symptoms in children aged 2–3 months.

6.4.2 Implementation of updated paediatric paracetamol dosing

The new dosage instructions for paediatric paracetamol will be on products entering the market by the end of 2011. In the meantime, parents and carers should follow the advice currently on the packaging. There is no need to remove any products from shelves. The new packs will also be supplied with a suitable measuring device to assist accurate administration.

The updated dosing will apply equally to prescribed paracetamol for children, and the BNF will be updated accordingly.
The advice for healthcare professionals is as follows:

- Parents and carers should be advised to follow the advice on the packaging

- The new dosing will be supplied with a revised patient information leaflet and packaging (entering the market by end 2011)

- All products will be supplied with an administration device to ensure accurate administration.

Aspirin must not be given to children younger than 16 (12 is the advised age in the USA) due to the risk of Reyes syndrome, a rare but very significant condition with mortality of up to 50%.

Within Ambulance Service practice, there is limited experience of using NSAIDs in caring for children. Although the use of ibuprofen is approved and advocated in JRCALC guidelines, the East of England has not adopted ibuprofen into standard practice.[181] Ibuprofen is highly effective in reducing the incidence of post-traumatic inflammation, as well as pain of musculoskeletal origin and pain associated with growing and teething. The MHRA no longer advocate the alternate use of paracetamol and ibuprofen suspensions concurrently, citing a lack of evidence of effectively managing a feverish child and potential risk associated with over-medication.[182] Ibuprofen is available as a suspension or syrup and should be given up to a dose of 20 mg/kg/day. Diclofenac is available as a suppository (12.5 mg or 25 mg) for paediatric use and can be used as an effective medication for moderate to severe pain. The dosage can be up to 3 mg/kg/day.

6.5 Opioid analgesia

Opioids are safe and effective in managing pain in both children and adults. A primary concern among ambulance clinicians in the use of morphine in children is the risk of respiratory depression, especially when larger doses are administered. In addition to this, in the absence of oromorph, many clinicians are hesitant to attempt intravenous cannulation of children. Opiate pain relief in children, however, is not limited by any means to morphine and oromorph. Codeine phosphate is a highly effective opioid analgesic, which is easily administered orally, often in conjunction with paracetamol. It is quickly metabolised into morphine and creates a number of analgesic metabolites, which when combined with the antipyrexial and anti-inflammatory properties of paracetamol, prove to be a very useful pain managing tool.

Codeine is also produced as a subcutaneous or intramuscular injection, effective in managing pain in babies and children experiencing ongoing pain within a community setting. Codeine should not be administered intravenously as it is strongly associated with severe acute hypotension and incidences of apnoea, especially in children.

Pain relief in the elderly

Lucas Hawkes-Frost and Tracy Nicholls

Summary

- The aging process – assessment of elderly patients is seen to be difficult by a great many clinicians, due to hearing, speech and cognitive impairments.

- Effects of pain relief on the elderly – changes in the physiology, endocrine and organ function in older patients, mean analgesic drugs are often poorly absorbed or ineffectively metabolised, leading to complications involving poor drug function, poor clearance and, ultimately, ineffective pain relief or unacceptable side effects.

- Hepatic and renal problems – a reduction in hepatic blood flow means a decrease in the metabolism of drugs. Morphine will primarily be cleared by the kidneys so, combined with the slower liver metabolism, this can result in an elderly patient having a higher potency of the opiate and possibly having the effects lasting for a longer period of time than anticipated.

7.1 The aging process

In the field of prehospital emergency care, the elderly population represents a significant majority of patient contacts during routine day-to-day operations. Clinically, elderly patients present special problems in the provision of analgesia. Difficulty with communication is a pervasive challenge with patients suffering from various presentations of dementia, as well as challenges posed by alterations in physiology in older patients. Assessment of elderly patients is seen to be difficult by a great many clinicians, with hearing, speech and cognitive impairments often affecting a clinician's ability to assess and accurately diagnose pain and discomfort. Indeed the provision of pain relief in the elderly patient is often a process fraught with difficulty, requiring a great deal of experience, intuition and estimation of a patient's presenting condition to correctly assess, identify and manage pain. Entonox can be poorly received due to dentition changes and the inability to take long, deep breaths, and this often leaves the elderly patient feeling nauseous.

Generally, elderly patients report pain significantly less frequently and request smaller doses of analgesic drugs to achieve what they describe as adequate pain relief. In the UK, elderly patients, especially those with dementia, receive up to 50% less analgesia than younger patients and those without symptoms of dementia.

The process of assessing pain in elderly patients should be virtually indistinguishable from that utilised in the assessment of a young adult, utilising numerical or pictorial/graphic pain assessment scales. However, in cases where a patient is suspected of suffering a degree of impaired higher intellectual function, clinicians must utilise alternative means of pain assessment including observational techniques such as the Abbey Pain Scale.

7.2 Effects of pain relief in the elderly

Owing to changes in the physiology, endocrine function and organ function in older patients, analgesic drugs are often poorly absorbed or ineffectively metabolised, leading to complications involving poor drug function, poor clearance and, ultimately, ineffective pain relief or unacceptable side effects. For example, a number of pharmacokinetic studies have been conducted in patients with a wide range in renal functionality, all receiving continuous intravenous infusion with morphine.[174] After researchers corrected their data for the morphine blood/plasma concentration ratio of 1.1 determined in humans,[183] it was observed that an accumulation of morphine metabolites proved a significant correlation between the half-life of certain morphine metabolites and the plasma concentration of urea in patients with renal failure.

Furthermore, it was observed that as creatinine clearance decreased in patients taking oral doses of morphine, the plasma concentration of two primary metabolites increased relatively to the plasma concentration of morphine. Following the administration of a metabolite of morphine, namely morphine-6-gluconuride, to two patients, one with normal and the other with impaired renal function, Osborne et al observed that the plasma clearance of that specific metabolite was closely linked to the excretion of creatinine.[183] The results of numerous studies have suggested strongly a significant link between the renal excretion and plasma clearance of morphine, its metabolites and renal creatinine. Any excessive use of opiates can worsen the already compromised renal function in the elderly.

7.3 Hepatic and renal problems

Opiates are absorbed in the gut and have a high first pass rate in the liver. They are then excreted through bile into faecal matter and into urine via the kidneys. The elderly patient has a decreased gastrointestinal transit time and an increased gastric pH level. They tend to have an increase in adipose tissue, decreased body mass and decreased total water content which results in opiates taking more time to be eliminated. Also, a reduction in hepatic blood flow means a decrease in the metabolism of drugs. Morphine will primarily be cleared by the kidneys so, combined with the slower liver metabolism, this can cause an elderly patient to have a higher potency of the opiate. Furthermore, it is possible that the effects will last for a longer period of time than anticipated.

It has been established that, when administered to elderly patients, analgesic drugs may not be absorbed well or metabolised efficiently. In terms of clinical practice, the process of dosing drugs such as NSAIDs and opioids should be reduced overall owing to this decrease in liver metabolism and renal function. In addition to this, the phenomenon of polypharmacy should be considered, as elderly patients, who are more likely to be receiving more than one drug for underlying medical conditions, are at significantly increased risk of drug interaction and paradoxical effects.

It is worth remembering that elderly patients may be particularly sensitive to opioid analgesia and are certainly more prone to unwanted side effects such as confusion, sedation and respiratory depression. As discussed previously, changes in both hepatic and renal function necessitate overall lower doses of opioids, which will potentially have a longer length of action. In clinical practice, especially in the context of the ambulance service, only one opioid drug should be used at a time to achieve effective pain relief, instead choosing a different drug group to complement an analgesic plan, for example, codeine and paracetamol.

In general practice, an elderly patient should receive an initial dose of approximately half the normal adult dose, especially if the drug is administered intravenously. From there, small maintenance doses should be given regularly to anticipate pain where appropriate.

When handing over patients to hospitals, care should be taken to explain the dose and rationale for the analgesia given, and concerns regarding renal function should be well documented. Elderly patients with acute pain may still require a reasonably high initial dose in the prehospital setting, and hospitals will need to take this into account and adjust subsequent doses and dosing intervals to accommodate this.

Pain and dementia

Michael Collins and Suzanne Lillington

Summary

- The ability to respond to pain – as dementia progresses, the ability to respond to pain becomes more impaired. It would appear that in advanced dementia the threshold at which the pain is recognised is increased.[187]

- Communication issues – cognitive impairment may prevent a patient communicating their needs as clearly as those patients without dementia. This can create huge barriers between patient and clinician, evident particularly during history taking and assessing pain levels, leading to a possible inaccurate conclusion and poorly managed pain.

- Abbey pain scale – the Abbey pain scale is one tool which may be of particular use in the prehospital setting. This one-page assessment tool uses non-verbal observation cues to ascertain the level of pain. The scale can be used as an assessment tool before intervention, such as pain relief, and afterwards, as a measure of effectiveness and success.

8.1 The ability to respond to pain

Managing pain in patients with dementia poses certain challenges. This is largely due to the obstacles around pain assessment and the specific neurodegenerative changes along pain pathways.

A question that seems to frequently arise is: 'Do patients with dementia feel pain similarly to those without dementia?' This is an important question to consider especially for clinicians assessing these patients. The answer is: yes they do! However, what often changes is the way the pain is presented and communicated by the patient to the clinician.

It is important to have an awareness of the changes within the brain caused by the different types of dementia, and the experiences of pain as a result of these. Different types of dementia may determine a different pain effect. For example, the pathophysiology of the brain in Alzheimer's disease is different from vascular dementia, or frontal temporal dementia.

Benedetti et al observed that in Alzheimer's disease the pain threshold did not differ from those without dementia, but the pain tolerance was increased.[207] The pain and discomfort was tolerated, before withdrawal from the painful source.

> As dementia progresses, the ability to respond to pain becomes more impaired. It would appear that in advanced dementia the threshold at which the pain is recognised is increased .[187]

8.2 Communication issues

A cognitive impairment may prevent a patient communicating their needs as clearly as those without dementia. This can create huge barriers between patient and clinician, evident particularly during history taking and assessing pain levels, leading to a possible inaccurate conclusion and poorly managed pain as a result. Horgas and Tsai evidenced in their report that doctors prescribed less analgesia for nursing home residents who were cognitively impaired than those with normal cognition.[208] Also those with dementia were given less nurse initiated pain relief.

This is a topic that has been in the spotlight for some time across the health service. Patients with dementia are often unable to describe their pain for many reasons, including communication and speech problems and are therefore frequently under-diagnosed and their pain will not be in-adequately addressed. Clinicians in the prehospital setting frequently find themselves assessing frail patients with dementia who may have frequent falls and musculoskeletal pain and mobility problems as a result, yet feel unable to ascertain the true level of pain which the patient is experiencing.

8.3 Abbey pain scale

An adequate tool for assessing patients with dementia is essential to ensure the optimum level of care is given to this patient group. Various assessment tools are available to assist with this complicated assessment.

The Abbey Pain Scale (see Chapter 5) is one such tool that may be of particular use in the prehospital setting. This one-page assessment tool uses non-verbal observation cues to ascertain the level of pain. The scale can be used as an assessment tool before intervention, such as pain relief, and afterwards, as a measure of effectiveness and success. A&E departments in England are beginning to use this tool to improve clinicians' recognition of pain levels in patients with dementia. Ambulance clinicians are encouraged to adopt the Abbey Scale as an aide memoir along with JRCALC guidelines[181] and other pathways that can be easily referenced. It can be used alongside any capacity assessments that are undertaken and promotes acting in the patient's best interest.

Pain management in patients with dementia is a critical issue. Despite considerable research, reports and studies, their pain remains under-recognised and misunderstood, often leading to poor assessment and inadequate treatment as a consequence.

8.4 Case study

A paramedic recently attended to a lady who had fallen in her warden-controlled flat and been discovered shortly after by her neighbour. The lady was in her 80s and the neighbour informed the crew that she often got confused; on examination she had an obvious deformity to her left wrist. She did appear to be confused and on further investigation it was concluded that she was suffering from mild dementia.

The paramedic noticed that the patient seemed quite agitated and kept looking at her injured wrist and rubbing it as if she was trying to 'rub it better'. The affected wrist was immobilised in a triangular bandage. Despite her obvious confusion she was able to tell the crew her personal details and seemed to have some understanding of what was going on. The paramedic concluded that the manner of the patient's actions were such that she was believed to be in pain. It was also decided that despite her understanding of simple issues, there was doubt that she would have enough understanding to adequately self-administer entonox to a level which would ease her pain.

The paramedic then asked if her wrist was painful to which she replied it was. She was asked if she would like an injection to help her with the pain; again, she replied yes. The crew decided to increase her pain relief and the paramedic cannulated the patient and slowly administered 2.5 mg of morphine followed by metaclopramide, as per the JRCALC guidelines. This was so that, if required, she could have further morphine titrated until the pain became tolerable, at 1 mg aliquots. After about 10 minutes the crew noticed that the patient had stopped attempting to rub the injured wrist and had also become more at ease and was less agitated. When asked if the pain was getting any better, she replied that it was.

The paramedic reflected that he was able to do this with confidence thanks to the clinical summit he had recently attended and the presentation on pain management which was given and also due to the current professional update course which had also included assessment and treatment of patients with dementia.

End-of-life patients and their pain mangement

Andrea Charles and Tracy Nicholls

Summary

- Types of pain in cancer – 40% of the type of pain seen in cancer patients is neuropathic.

- Assessment of pain – careful questioning and communication is required to obtain a full history of the type, area and duration of pain. Once the pain has been assessed, a plan of action needs to be formulated. Prior to immediately looking at the pharmacological route we need to briefly consider all options.

- Alternative pain relief – cognitive activities like distraction techniques and relaxation can decrease pain perception.

- Anticipatory prescribing – these are a box of prescribed medications that are already in the house to be given. They are all given intra-muscularly (IM) or subcutaneously (SC) and dosage instructions are in the patient notes.

9.1 Types of pain

According to the National Council for Hospice and Specialist Palliative Care Services no patient should experience pain without receiving some help to reduce it.

The type of pain end-of-life patients suffer can differ from the normal type of pain experienced by others. Neuropathic pain accounts for 40% of cancer pain – this is pain caused by pathological changes in the nervous system. It is different from pain due to trauma as it is caused by damage to the nervous system. Neuropathic pain is commonly felt as a burning or stabbing sensation. These patients commonly suffer other medical problems, including falls and injuries that cause regular pain as well. An end-of-life patient can therefore suffer from acute and neuropathic pain simultaneously.

Pain management in end-of-life care is a clinical area in which the ambulance service could improve. Common reasons for poor pain management include inadequate pain assessment, fear of giving more medications on top of their own and the thought that being in pain may be 'normal' and has to be accepted for these patients.

End-of-life cancer patients often under-report their pain and don't report all their symptoms as they are worried about being labelled as a 'bad patient'. Pain may also influence mood, so prejudices should not be made if a patient appears to be detached or short tempered with family members or clinicians.

Pain is a subjective experience and so it can be hard to view it objectively. Pain assessment tools are one way of accomplishing this. These are especially relevant to patients who are unable to verbally communicate effectively, which may be due to nearing the end of life or dementia or other illness.

9.2 Assessment

How is pain currently assessed in these patients? Pain management at the end of life relies on accurate pain assessment. Careful questioning and communication is required to obtain a full history of the type, area and duration of pain. Once the pain has been assessed, a plan of action then needs to formulated. Prior to immediately looking at the pharmacological route we need to briefly consider all options, as shown in the therapeutic ladder for pain management in Figure 9.1.

There are of course other ways of managing pain without using drugs. Emotional aspects of the experience of pain, for example cognitive activities like distraction techniques and relaxation, can decrease pain perception and the provision of comfort is a primary intervention for the control of pain.[209]

From an ambulance service point of view these patients will often already have a multidisciplinary team assigned to them including carers, district nurses, Macmillan nurses, physiotherapists, occupational therapists and doctors, just to name a few. It can often be hard to make sense of the care notes and establish who should be doing what.

Family members often have high expectations of the ambulance service and expect us as an agency to fully understand a vast number of medical illnesses and know how to treat them effectively (which isn't always the case, especially with rare illnesses –remember to be professional and to instill confidence in the patient).

One of the concerns often raised by ambulance staff is centred on how to know which of the analgesic drugs can be given on top of a patient's current medication. Clinical advice for clinicians can give crews support in this often confusing area.

9.3 Alternatives for pain relief

Many end-of-life patients will already be receiving pain relief medication. Gabapentin is often given to control neuropathic pain. Various patches, including oromorph, fentanyl lollies and towards the very end of life, a syringe driver may administer strong opioids.

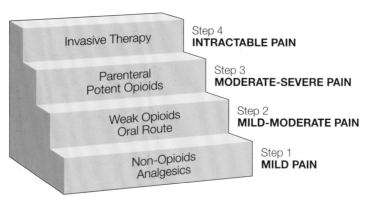

Figure 9.1 Therapeutic ladder for pain management in terminally ill patients.

Currently, options include entonox, oromorph, IV morphine and also to administer the anticipatory drugs the patient already has prescribed (following clinical advice if necessary). Entonox takes some effort on the patient's part to administer and is often not understood or the patients are simply too weak to operate it. Anecdotally, there is often a reluctance (especially in the elderly) to accept morphine as many people associate morphine with addiction, loss of control and even death. These cases are when communication becomes crucially important. IV interventions are often declined by end of life patients as well and often they may have a poor vasculature which makes cannulation very hard – the last thing they need is for someone to have many attempts to gain IV access. In these occasions oromorph may be more appropriate and worth considering.

Some patients may have their own fentanyl lollipops, which are given for breakthrough pain. They were highly publicised when the *Daily Mail* printed pictures of Jade Goody sucking them on discharge from hospital appointments.[184] Fentanyl is a very strong analgesic, and in the lollipop form can work within 15 minutes. Fentanyl patches can take 24 hours to reach full potential but will continue to provide pain relief for up to 72 hours. The lolly form is non-invasive and little effort is required by the patient and hence they may be a possibility for the ambulance services to use in the future, if the laws around possession of fentanyl should change.

9.4 Anticipatory prescribing

In addition, remember the clinical ability that now allows ambulance staff (under GP/clinical advice) to administer the patients with anticipatory drugs. These are a box of prescribed medications that are already in the house to be given. They are all given IM or SC and dosage instructions are in the patient notes. These drugs are often the key in making end-of-life patients comfortable, helping them to reduce their pain and allowing them to maintain their dignity.

In conclusion we should acknowledge that pain is whatever the sufferer says it is. We need to make sure we undertake a full assessment and understand the symptoms, then decide with the patient and/or their relatives the best course of action in order to make these patients comfortable and to reduce their pain where possible. This will require an up-to-date knowledge of all the internal and external resources available in our working area to ensure these patients have the best outcome during a time that may be deeply distressing for the patient and their families.

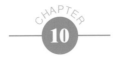

Active cooling and cryotherapy as pain relief

Lucas Hawkes-Frost

Summary

- 'RICE' – the active cooling of an injured area of soft tissue or a joint in the hope that it will reduce swelling, inflammation and ultimately pain.

- Nerve conduction velocity – potential mechanisms by which analgesic effects may be brought about through the active reduction of temperature in local areas of soft tissue, postulating that this specific intervention acts through reducing nerve conduction velocity (NCV).

10.1 'RICE'

All clinical staff within the realm of prehospital care are familiar with the acronym 'RICE', referring to the management of soft tissue and joint injuries. One key component of 'RICE' is the active cooling of an injured area of soft tissue or a joint in the hope that it will reduce swelling, inflammation and ultimately pain. Many conflicting opinions persist on the value of such activities in reducing pain. As a publically accountable organisation, the Ambulance Service must demonstrate that advice and clinical care provided are based on sound clinical evidence. What, then, is the evidence to support or indeed to discount the value of cooling and cryotherapy, especially in the prehospital arena and particularly in the immediate aftermath of the injury or insult dealt to the patient? In their article, Algafly and George laid out convincing data in support of the position that cryotherapy or active cooling of an injured site is an effective, inexpensive and simple intervention for pain management.[154, 155]

10.2 Nerve conduction velocity

Their study has suggested a number of potential mechanisms by which analgesic effects may be brought about through the active reduction of temperature in local areas of soft tissue, postulating that this specific intervention acts through reducing nerve conduction velocity (NCV).

Research suggests that NCV is significantly and progressively reduced in direct relation with skin temperature at the ankle during the application of cryotherapy. In addition to reductions in observed NCV, Algafly and George further observed significant increases in individual pain thresholds and pain tolerances at two assessment sites on the ankle, served by the same nerve. Their study suggests that specifically, a reduction in skin temperature to 10°C resulted in an average reduction of 33% in NCV. This reduction in NCV equates to a 0.4 m/s decrease in sensory NVC for each 1°C fall in skin temperature assuming the experiment begins with a skin temperature of around 31°C.

Chesterton et al[154] report that by reducing the skin temperature 10–13.5°C, NCV was reduced by approximately 10% compared with the 17% reduction in NCV at 15°C and the 33% reduction in NCV reduction at 10°C in the Algafly and George study.

Although no consensus exists around the physiological rationale for the functional changes in neurophysiology during cryotherapy, it is thought that temperature fluctuation may affect ionic exchange between Ca^{2+} and Na^+ in nociceptive afferent neurones.

Reid et al observed in their study that when cooled to physiologically low temperatures, friction increased between Ca^{2+} ions and the cellular 'gates' responsible for controlling the influx and outflow of calcium ions from the neurone, effectively slowing the process of generating action potentials and ultimately reducing nerve activity.[155]

In the same study, it was noted that, associated with the drop in NCV, there was a concomitant increase in patient pain threshold and pain tolerance which appeared to be linked to skin temperature reduction. It is interesting to note that in a certain study, investigators observe that during exposure to a cold environment (19°C) for around 30 mins, plasma endorphin levels doubled. This increase in plasma concentrations of endorphins, a key neurotransmitter responsible for pleasure, should affect the patient systemically and increase the pain threshold and tolerance throughout the body.

Ultimately, the evidence supporting the use of active cooling as a means of relieving pain is intriguing, revealing that cooling at the ankle and indeed other joints and soft tissue sites around the body may result in an increased pain tolerance and pain threshold both at the site of ice application and cooling and at sites distal to cooling but still innervated by a common nerve. In the context of prehospital emergency care, it would seem prudent to suggest that the application of active cooling has a place in clinical practice extending beyond the scope of patients currently receiving therapies actively designed to reduce skin temperature, namely in the treatment of burns.

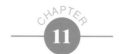

What can specialist paramedics do for patients in pain?

Mark Eardley

Summary

- Introduction – opioids remain the mainstay of treatment for moderate to severe nociceptive pain, with morphine remaining the most widely used opiate in its management; however, it is not always the case that morphine is the most suitable or effective analgesia for some pain states.

- Analgesics – two main advantages to having a wider analgesic armamentarium are being able to select a single analgesic alternative to morphine in appropriate circumstances and being able to use a rational multimodal analgesic approach to pain management.

- Local anaesthetics – a preparation of 1% lidocaine local anaesthetic is carried by specialist paramedics. Its primary indication is to facilitate examination, cleansing and closure of wounds.

- NSAIDs – paracetamol, when combined with NSAIDs, was found to have greater analgesic efficacy than paracetamol alone.

- Paracetamol – also an effective adjunct to opioids analgesia, opioid requirements being reduced by 20–30% when combined with a regular regimen of oral or rectal paracetamol, and is more effective when combined with an opioid or NSAID.

- Steroids – there is evidence that when added to acyclovir, prednisolone can help reduce the acute phase pain of herpes zoster.

11.1 Introduction

Although opioids remain the mainstay of treatment for moderate to severe nociceptive pain, with morphine remaining the most widely used opiate in its management, it is not always the case that morphine is the most suitable or effective analgesia for some pain states.[188]

Specialist paramedics operating within Ambulance Trusts have undergone training and education in primary care assessment and management models, including using a wide range of pharmacological analgesics (based on the core competencies).[189]

Two main advantages to having a wider analgesic armamentarium are:

1. Being able to select a single analgesic alternative to morphine in appropriate circumstances.
2. Or, being able to use a rationale multimodal analgesic approach to pain management.

Having training in primary care also exposes Specialist paramedics to patients who are experiencing chronic pain states, including neuropathic pain, where management may differ from patients in acute pain; and gaining experience in using an 'analgesic ladder' methodology, and use of biopsychosocial pain assessment models.

Last but not least, Specialist paramedics during out of hours have access to: GP colleagues who may be able to prescribe a wider range of analgesic agents under appropriate circumstances; hospital colleagues to discuss complicated or uncertain cases, where admission may be required either for pain management or further investigation of a patient's pain; and referral mechanisms to the patient's own GP for ongoing management where admission is not appropriate.

11.2 Analgesics

11.2.1 Acyclovir (anti-viral)

Oral medication available.

Indications: herpes zoster virus. If given within 72 hours of the herpes zoster rash appearing, it can shorten the duration of acute pain.[190]

Contraindications: patients under 16 years, known hypersensitivity to acyclovir, patients who are immunocompromised, pregnancy and breast-feeding, known renal impairment/on renal dialysis.

11.2.2 Anti-fungal (nystatin)

Oral medication available.

Indications: nystatin is used to treat oral candidiasis, which can be a painful and distressing condition (and is also used to treat fungal infections of the skin, mouth, vagina, and intestinal tract).

Contraindications: patients under 1 month, patients with a known hypersensitivity to nystatin.

11.2.3 Anti-spasmodic (hyoscine butylbromide)

Parenteral and oral anti-spasmodic medications are available.

Indications: spasm in the gastrointestinal tract or the genitourinary tract. It is also of particular benefit in inoperable malignant bowel obstruction patients who are suffering colicky abdominal pain.[191]

Contraindications: under 15 years for parental injection, under 6 years for oral medication; myasthenia gravis, megacolon, paralytic ileus, narrow angle glaucoma, pyloric stenosis, known hypersensitivity to hyoscine, urinary retention.

11.2.4 Co-codamol/codeine phosphate/dihydrocodeine

Oral medication available.

Indications: treatment of mild to moderate pain, and moderate to severe pain (depending on drug and preparation), in children over the age of 12 years.

Contraindications:

Codeine phosphate and dihydrocodeine – acute respiratory depression, acute alcoholism, head injury with the risk of raised intracranial pressure, acute asthma, hypersensitivity to codeine.

Co-codamol – acute respiratory depression, acute alcoholism, head injury with the risk of raised intracranial pressure, acute asthma, following biliary surgery, monoamine oxidise inhibitor therapy – concurrent or within 14 days, hypersensitivity to paracetamol or codeine.

11.2.5 Constipation pain medications (glycerin suppository, Relaxit® micro-enema)

Indications: to relieve constipation.

Contraindications:

Glycerin suppositories – intestinal obstruction.
Relaxit® micro-enema – children under the age of 3 years, patients with inflammatory bowel disease.

11.2.6 Gastrointestinal drugs: Gaviscon®/Peptac® (alginate reflux suppressant and antacid), Lansoprazole (proton pump inhibitor), Ranitidine (H2 receptor antagonist).

Oral medication available.

Indications: symptomatic relief of gastro-oesophageal reflux, dyspepsia characterised by pain, heartburn and epigastric discomfort.

Proton pump inhibitors also significantly reduce the incidences of non-steroidal anti-inflammatory drug induced peptic ulceration.[192]

Contraindications:

Gaviscon® – children under 12 years of age, hypersensitivity to active ingredients of Gaviscon®.

Peptac® – children under 6 years of age, hypersensitivity to active ingredients of Peptac®.

Lansoprazole – children under the age of 16 years, patients who are pregnant, known hypersensitivity to lansoprazole.

Ranitidine – known hypersensitivity to ranitidine, patients under the age of 16 years, pregnancy and breastfeeding, history of porphyria, patients who are HIV positive and are receiving Saquinavir.

11.3 Local anaesthetics

A preparation of 1% lidocaine local anaesthetic is carried by specialist paramedics. Its primary indication is to facilitate examination, cleansing and closure of wounds.

However, intradermal local infiltration with lidocaine has proven efficacy in reducing the pain of cannulation compared with entonox and freeze sprays.[193,194] Although topical local anaesthetic cream has proved successful, its average time of affect of 60 minutes makes its use impractical in the acute setting.

Lidocaine infiltration may, therefore, be appropriate and beneficial in patients who require cannulation for opioids analgesia but are apprehensive of venepuncture (e.g. children).

It should be borne in mind that local anaesthetic infiltration will sting but probably not as much as cannulation with a larger bore cannula.

(Of interest are gas pressure syringes, which provide local infiltration of lidocaine prior to venepuncture, that have been used with good efficacy, but with varying degrees of comfort during administration.[195,196] These are not currently used in UK ambulance trusts.)

The intradermal injection of local anaesthetic, however, can be made more comfortable by warming the local anaesthetic prior to use.[197]

11.3.1 Migraine medication (rizatriptan)

Oral medication available.

Indications: for the relief of an acute migraine attack in patients over the age of 18 years. They are effective in migraine attacks which have led to severe pain and disability where 'simple analgesia' has failed.[198]

Contraindications: adults less than 18 years old and children, hypersensitivity to rizatriptan, concurrent administration of a monoamine oxidase inhibitor (MAOI) or within 2 weeks of stopping a MAOI, patients with severe hepatic or renal insufficiency, patients who have had a previous stroke or TIA, severe hypertension or untreated mild hypertension, established coronary artery disease, peripheral vascular disease, on other similar medications, e.g. ergometrine, patients who have taken propranolol less than 2 hours previously, patients who have taken any of the 'triptan' group of medications in the past 24 hours.

11.3.2 Muscle relaxants (diazepam)

Oral medication available.

Indications: in the context of analgesia – for the treatment of acute muscle spasm in patients over the age of 16 years.

Diazepam is not recommended for routine use, due to its side effect profile; however, it can be added onto other medications where its benefits are believed to outweigh any side effects.[199]

Contraindications: in the context of analgesia – muscle spasm in patients under the age of 16 years, patients known to be hypersensitive to benzodiazepines, patients who are pregnant or breastfeeding.

11.4 Non-steroidal anti-inflammatory drugs (diclofenac and ibuprofen)

Diclofenac: oral, rectal and injectable medications available.
Ibuprofen: oral medications available.

Indications:

Diclofenac – pain and inflammation in acute musculoskeletal disorders, pain due to renal colic, acute dental problems.

Ibuprofen: pain and inflammation in acute musculoskeletal disorders, as an antipyretic medication, for post immunisation fever control.

Paracetamol, when combined with NSAIDs, was found to have greater analgesic efficacy than paracetamol alone.[200]

Ibuprofen has the least adverse effects of all the NSAIDs.[201]

There is little evidence to recommend any one particular NSAID over another[202] but NSAIDs are best used as part of multimodal analgesia along with paracetamol and/or opiates.

Parenteral diclofenac is as effective as parenteral opioids in the treatment of biliary colic.[203]

NSAIDs reduce requirements for rescue analgesia and produce less vomiting than opioids in renal colic.[204]

Contraindications:

Diclofenac – children under the age of 16 years, adults with active or suspected gastrointestinal ulcers or bleeding, patients who are sensitive to diclofenac/aspirin/other NSAIDS, asthmatics who have never used an NSAID before or have severe asthma or had worsening of asthma symptoms after previous use, patients who have severe heart failure, known pregnancy, patients on concurrent anticoagulants (warfarin, heparin, clopidogrel, aspirin, or other NSAID), porphyria.

In addition contraindicated for injection only: patients on mannitol, patients on concomitant NSAIDS or anti-coagulants, a history of confirmed or suspected cerebro-vascular bleeding, patients with known severe renal impairment, hypovolaemia, dehydration.

Ibuprofen – known hypersensitivity to aspirin, ibuprofen, or other NSAID; children under 7 kg, pregnancy, current or previous history of dyspepsia or peptic ulceration, asthmatics who have never used an NSAID before or have severe asthma or had worsening of asthma symptoms after previous use, patients on concurrent anticoagulants, patients taking tacrolimus (*an immunosuppressive drug taken after organ transplantation), lithium (mood stabiliser), methotrexate (a chemotherapy drug), ciclosporin ((cyclosporine) an immunosuppressant drug taken for ulcerative colitis), patients with known severe cardiac disease, heart failure, oedema, hypertension or renal impairment.*

11.5 Paracetamol

Oral or rectal medication available.

Indications: for the treatment of mild to moderate pain, and pyrexia in adults and children over 3 months. Post immunisation vaccination pyrexia in infants under 3 months.

Paracetamol is also an effective adjunct to opioid analgesia, opioid requirements being reduced by 20–30% when combined with a regular regimen of oral or rectal paracetamol, and is more effective when combined with an opioid or NSAID.[200]

Contraindications: known hypersensitivity to paracetamol, patients with known alcohol dependency, severe liver disease, children under 3 months old (except for post vaccination pyrexia), patients who have taken paracetamol containing products within the previous 4 hours, patients who have taken 4 or more doses of paracetamol within the previous 24 hours.

11.6 Steroids (prednisolone)

Oral medication available.

Indications: in the context of analgesia – for the treatment of suspected temporal arteritis.

There is evidence that when added to acyclovir, prednisolone can help reduce the acute phase pain of herpes zoster.[205]

Contraindications: in the context of temporal arteritis – patients under the age of 20 years, known hypersensitivity to prednisolone.

Note: all contraindications as per Patient Group Directions within the East of England Ambulance Service NHS Trust.

Specialist paramedics and critical care

Tim Hayes, Daimon Wheddon and Ashley Richardson

Summary

- Paracetamol – an analgesic drug with anti-pyretic properties, which may be provided to patients in moderate to severe pain.

- Ketamine – a PCP derivative providing specific significant anaesthetic, analgesic and amnesic properties with minimal effects on respiratory centre. It interacts at the NMDA receptor complex promoting neurotransmitter inhibition and affecting opioid receptors, which account for analgesic effect. NMDA excitatory synaptic transmitters in the CNS allow sodium, calcium and potassium to flow into and out of the cells. The NMDA agonist mimics the action of the neurotransmitter glutamate on NMDA receptors.

- Fentanyl – a potent opiate analgesic (approximately 100 times more potent than morphine sulphate). It is both rapid in onset and short in duration of action.

- Diamorphine – a strong opioid drug that works as an agonist to mu receptors. It can be given intranasally and so is an alternative analgesic agent available for children where gaining IV access is either impossible or will cause unnecessary distress.

- Nerve blocks – subcutaneous injections of a local anaesthetic into nerves can be used to provide effective analgesia to specific body parts. This would be commonly used to provide pain relief to a hand, foot or section of the thigh. This can be useful, for example, where that body part is trapped in machinery and needs to be manipulated to allow extrication and where sedation is inappropriate, e.g. if the patient cannot be laid down.

The provision of enhanced medical care and prehospital critical care by or to the Trust, is currently delivered in a number of ways and by a number of providers. These providers are generally split into two categories: Level 3 – 'Anaesthetic' capable, which is delivered by a specialist physician or medical team; or Level 2 – 'Sub-anaesthetic' capable, which is delivered by a specialist paramedic (critical care) or other physician (i.e. BASICs doctor).

With regard to additional pain management options and strategies, this will depend on the level and capability of the provider. Capability may be affected by training, experience, logistics or legislation.

12.1 Specialist physician/medical team

A specialist physician or a medical team (physician/paramedic) can offer a wide range of pain management interventions. With regards to non-pharmacological interventions the medical team can obviously utilise the full range of splinting mechanisms and apply all psychological aspects of pain management as per any other healthcare professional.

Pharmacological analgesia options for a specialist physician or a medical team is not limited by legislation (due to the medico-legal situation with regards to a physician) though analgesia options are limited through logistics (i.e. what is carried by those providers). Most providers will utilise a similar skill set although there may be some variance.

The pain management options available to prehospital medical teams (e.g. doctor/paramedic helicopter teams and BASICS schemes) include paracetamol, ketamine, diamorphine, fentanyl, lidocaine and nerve blocks.

12.1.1 Paracetamol given by IV infusion

This drug is available to specialist paramedics (critical care) as an alternative to morphine administration for moderate to severe pain in adults and children. It is given by IV infusion over a period of 15 minutes. It may be of use if morphine is contraindicated, e.g. if the patient is too hypotensive to allow safe administration.

Paracetamol is an analgesic drug with anti-pyretic properties, which may be provided to patients in moderate to severe pain. The main action of paracetamol is the inhibition of cyclo-oxygenase (COX); it more specifically inhibits COX-2. Paracetamol reduces the amount of prostaglandins and therefore allows for reducing the patient's temperature. Paracetamol also inhibits the activation of nociceptors (pain receptors); these would normally be activated by anandamide. The metabolised form of paracetamol (AM404) inhibits the uptake of anandamide affording its analgesic properties.

At present IV paracetamol is the only addition to the analgesic formulary offered by paramedics; this may change in the event of legislation changes within the UK.

12.1.2 Ketamine

Ketamine is a PCP derivative providing specific significant anaesthetic, analgesic and amnesic properties with minimal effects on the respiratory centre. It interacts at the NMDA receptor complex promoting neuro-transmitter inhibition and affecting opioid receptors, which account for the analgesic effect. NMDA excitatory synaptic transmitters in the CNS allow sodium, calcium and potassium to flow in and out of the cells. The NMDA agonist mimics the action of the neurotransmitter glutamate on NMDA receptors.

Although ketamine increases pulse rate, cardiac output, blood pressure and muscle tone by direct cardiovascular system stimulation (caution in isolated head injury), it also has the ability to reduce blood pressure and cardiac output, especially in shocked patients.

Ketamine also has a bronchodilator effect and is safe for use with asthmatics. It is metabolised within the liver and excreted via the kidneys.

Ketamine is a drug that can cause analgesia in small doses. It causes less hypotension than morphine and so can be considered for use in situations where the patient is too cardiovascularly unstable to allow morphine administration; or where morphine has already been given and further analgesia is required.

In slightly larger doses, ketamine moves from providing analgesia to providing sedation. Sedation using ketamine or a combination of morphine and midazolam aims to sedate the patient (causing a reduction in their level of consciousness so that they are rousable but unaware of pain). For this to occur full monitoring must be used and the patient must be in a situation where they can be laid flat and airway management can take place. The sedation will usually be given in order for a procedure to take place that would cause pain, e.g. extrication from a vehicle where the patient's broken limbs must be manipulated to achieve this; or realignment of a fractured limb. Once the procedure has been undertaken sedation will usually be allowed to wear off. There are other situations where sedation may be used to gain control of combative patients but these are outside the scope of this chapter.

12.1.3 Intranasal diamorphine for analgesia in children

Diamorphine is a strong opioid drug that works as an agonist to mu receptors and can be given intranasally. Hence, it is an alternative analgesic agent available for children where gaining IV access is either impossible or will cause unnecessary distress. With the re-introduction of oromorph into paramedic practice it is likely that intranasal diamorphine will be rarely required, though its onset of action is quicker than oromorph.

12.1.4 Fentanyl

Fentanyl is a potent opiate analgesic (approximately 100 times more potent than morphine sulphate). It is both rapid in onset and short in duration of action. In UK prehospital practice fentanyl is most commonly used in the pre-treatment phase prior to some anaesthetic cases but can be used as an effective analgesic.

12.1.5 Lidocaine

Lidocaine is a class 1b anti-arrhythmic drug. This classification of anti-arrhythmic drugs block sodium channels, which prevents action potentials, thereby effecting nervous transmission. Lidocaine is used in the pre-hospital environment to provide local anaesthesia or regional nerve blocks. These are particularly effective in femoral shaft fractures and trapped extremities.

12.1.6 Nerve blocks using lidocaine or similar local anaesthetic drugs

A nerve block is an anaesthetic or anti-inflammatory injection targeted towards a certain nerve, or group of nerves to treat pain. The purpose of this is to 'switch off' pain signals from a specific area of the body.

Subcutaneous injections of a local anaesthetic into nerves can be used to provide effective analgesia to specific body parts. This would be commonly used to provide pain relief to a hand, foot or section of the thigh. This can be useful, for example, where that body part is trapped in machinery and needs to be manipulated to allow extrication and where sedation is inappropriate, e.g. if the patient cannot be laid down.

Figures 12.1a and 12.1b illustrate the underlying structures when looking to provide a femoral nerve block and the technique for undertaking this procedure. This is a significant step towards enhanced patient care and pain alleviation at the point of injury.

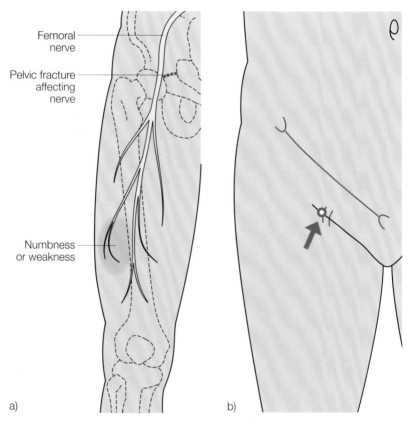

Femoral nerve

Pelvic fracture affecting nerve

Numbness or weakness

a)

b)

Figure 12.1a and 12.1b a) The underlying physiology of the femoral nerve; b) The site for insertion of the femoral nerve block.

Other nerve blocks can include ring, ulnar and median (Figure 12.2).

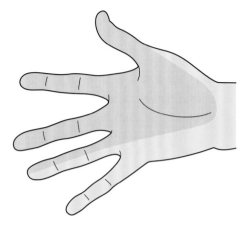

Figure 12.2 Area affected following a median nerve block.

It is important to remember that procedural sedation does not necessarily provide analgesia to a patient; this will depend on the agent used. For example, the most commonly used sedative agents, benzodiazepines (midazolam, diazepam) do not have any analgesic properties and it is therefore important to consider and use analgesics in the care of these patients.

12.2 Non-anaesthetic capable physician

There is currently no standardised skill set for these doctors and therefore pain management options may vary from provider to provider.

12.3 The specialist paramedic (critical care)

The specialist paramedic (critical care) role within prehospital care works as either an autonomous practitioner or as part of a physician/paramedic medical team. Dependent on their working role, the specialist paramedic (critical care) has various different treatment options available for the management of pain; the enhanced team role is discussed above. It is important to remember the same principles remain in place as for all other clinical grades and as such pain management encapsulates both non-pharmacological management and pharmacological management of pain. Autonomous practice for the specialist paramedic (critical care) allows care of a critically ill or injured patient to sub-anaesthetic level. As an autonomous practitioner the specialist paramedic (critical care) has options available to them, although currently the law does not allow for paramedics to possess or supply ketamine for patients who may need its therapeutic benefits.

Specialist paramedics (critical care) can provide all forms of splinting as per other clinical grades, although these also include:

- SAM pelvic splint allows for stabilisation of pelvic fractures; it works by providing equal force around the pelvis and if applied correctly (over the greater trocanters) affords stability of the pelvis.

- Kendrick Traction Device (KTD) is an alternative traction splint (similar to that of the Sagar traction splint), though can be used in a greater proportion of patients. There is one size of KTD that can be modified to allow for use in both adult and paediatric patients. The KTD can also be used in patients with suspected pelvic fracture; this is because they do not apply traction through the pelvis (unlike the Sagar traction splint).

It is important to remember that (dependent on the drug used) interventions such as procedural sedation and prehospital emergency anaesthesia do not provide analgesia to a patient. It is therefore important to consider and use analgesics in the care of these patients.

Critical care is constantly changing and developing to meet the needs of patients. With this changing environment the care options available to the specialist paramedic (critical care) and the physician/paramedic medical teams are constantly evolving.

Reassurance

Lucas Hawkes-Frost

Summary

- What is reassurance and who are we reassuring? – the patient can be said to have been reassured only if the 'reassurance' provided achieves an outcome of changing the patient's behaviour, understanding or outlook on their condition or the situation at hand.

Reassurance is an interventional technique thought by many to improve the efficacy of pain relief through achieving a reduction in anxiety and fear being experienced by a patient in pain. In practice, however, the notion of giving reassurance to a patient is an ambiguous concept. One clinician's outlook on what constitutes reassurance may be squarely at odds with a patient's expectations or personal needs. Indeed, many ambulance service staff will remember well the ubiquitous 'provide reassurance' catch-all answer on IHCD short answer question papers; indeed JRCALC give frequent reference to the importance of providing reassurance. Fundamentally, what is reassurance, and how should prehospital clinical staff structure this emotional support to best benefit their patients? Reassurance is generally recommended as being beneficial owing to the 'implicit conceptualisation model', which assumes that information provided to patients pertaining to their presenting medical condition is a means of empowering them in the process of the provision of healthcare. In addition to this, it is widely accepted that if a clinician is able to correct inaccurate beliefs the patient may hold, the associated fear based on those beliefs will be addressed simultaneously. Ultimately, correcting mistaken beliefs should reduce anxiety, which in turn should allow the patient to function in a more empowered and informed way. However, according to Linton et al, in their review published in Pain, the concept of the provision of reassurance in pursuit of pain management has very little evidence to support it and certainly fails to appreciate the complex nature of pain and the ways in which patients experience pain.[148]

In their paper, Linton et al posit that the actual act of providing reassurance is a complex series of processes requiring a great deal of nuanced interaction and interpersonal communication, necessitating an intimate knowledge, by both parties, of the experience, thoughts and emotions the patient is experiencing, which may be dynamic and changeable in nature. This discourse depends largely on the thoughts and beliefs of the patient and the clinician. The patient can be said to have been reassured only if the 'reassurance' provided achieves an outcome of changing the patient's behaviour, understanding or outlook on their condition or the situation at hand.

It would seem, then, that the glib statement 'provide reassurance' is not as straightforward as could easily be assumed on a cursory glance. The method of providing reassurance is squarely the responsibility of the clinician and requires them to behave in such a way as to facilitate the communication of information, instruction and persuasion.

Ambulance Service staff, through experience and exposure, are often thought and said, anecdotally, to have great powers of persuasion. This is again mentioned in the JRCALC guidelines issued to clinicians.[181] Within ambulance operations, reassurance is often given in the form of suggested corrective information, and often involves the explanation of physical explanations, mitigation of assessment results, or indeed minimalisation of prognosis.

Although the content of this information sharing is most often accurate, in no way does it guarantee that a patient will respond to them individually or as a professional with reduced anxiety or changed outlook. For example, evidence mentioned in the study by Linton asserts that when a clinician provides information that does not specifically address the concerns of the patient, or in any unintentional way diminishes the seriousness with which the patient views their condition ('you'll be fine'), they often respond by elaborating or insisting on the nature and severity of their symptoms more vigorously.[148] In the course of the study, it was discovered that reassurance was generally only accepted when given alongside an explanation that was relevant and went some way to addressing the patient's concerns and effectively established links between physical and psychological aspects of their presenting condition. The provision of vague platitudes may therefore be of little value, and constitute a poor experience for both the clinician and the patient.

Paradoxically, Linton et al cite studies which have demonstrated convincingly that providing reassurance linked to stressing the clinical insignificance of a patient's condition can actually have the effect of increasing the patient's anxiety and perceptions of impending peril, potentially increasing fear of future pain.[148] In addition to this, a number of studies have suggested that the provision of hollow reassurance, especially to patients suffering relatively mild conditions, may complicate matters by encouraging reassurance-seeking behaviour, such as requests for information from other health professionals and requests for tests and diagnostic procedures of little or no value to their presenting condition.[148] Although there seems to be little in the way of published evidence to suggest an intrinsic clinical value to reassurance; that is not to say that it is not a potentially important aspect of the clinician–patient relationship. Rather than encouraging lip service and reassurance, clinicians should concentrate on establishing a rapport and a trusting line of communication through which the patient feels confident in disclosing personal and at times sensitive information, and the clinician feels confident and comfortable asking the questions that need to be answered in the course of their patient assessment. In doing so, the ambulance service, as a clinical entity, can move away from advocating the provision of reassurance and move towards encouraging patients to take an active part in the management of their condition, especially when that condition involves pain. By communicating with patients in a manner that is empathetic and sympathetic to patients' anxieties and fears but does not seek to minimise the fear and discomfort they may be feeling, the clinician is bearing witness to the patient at a time when they may be at a particularly low ebb and be feeling especially vulnerable and frightened, thereby actively involving them in taking steps to manage their condition and treat their pain.

The provision of didactic information may go some way to reducing fear in some patients. However, direct attempts to influence thoughts and beliefs in a clinical setting, especially in an emergency, through the administration of reassurance in the form of dispassionate information sharing will almost certainly not be effective.

Ultimately, all health professionals, especially those working for agencies such as the ambulance service, where clinical situations are encountered immediately post insult or at the point of an exacerbation of an existing condition, have a responsibility to act in such a way as to provide empathy and enhance acceptance, rather than encourage patients to suppress fear and anxiety. Taking steps to involve patients in addressing their fears around pain is an effective and proactive way in which to reduce the development of worsened anxiety, avoidance and other counterproductive behaviours.

Conclusion

Lucas Hawkes-Frost and Tracy Nicholls

Pain control constitutes a significant and hugely important aspect of prehospital care and remains a primary reason for patient contacts in UK Ambulance Services. For too long, pain and, more importantly, the way we as prehospital clinicians manage pain, have fallen victim to myth and inappropriate prioritisation. Many patients may have suffered unnecessarily due to insufficient pain relief and an inability amongst the UK Ambulance Service system to adequately understand and address the pain a patient is feeling. The contribution that paramedics, EMTs, ECAs and volunteer staff have made and continue to make in the future are coalescing into a professional culture in which it is considered increasingly unreasonable to fail to treat pain. And the practice of doing so is seen as poor clinical care and unethical practice.

It is clear that there needs to be a wide range of pain relief available to staff to enable patients to receive adequate relief from their symptoms. The current availability of analgesia for mild to moderate pain relief is found to be lacking, as is analgesia for children. Some of this is based around education and a further development of the paramedic profession as a whole. The advent of specialist paramedics (ECPs) has seen a welcome addition to a wider formulary for the group of patients who experience moderate pain. However, the whole concept of the use of specialist paramedics is in its infancy and these paramedics are trying to find their way in a predominantly emergency care focused environment. The ability to give longer term pain relief with advice should not be underestimated and should be encouraged in order to provide a first class health service from our profession to our patients.

Pain in children needs closer consideration. The use of intranasal fentanyl is widely used in Australia by paramedics and is a development that would be received well within the UK. Alternatively, there may be other options to consider and we are currently exploring those. However, this will mean a change in the law around possession and supply that can only come through government. Also, the consideration of the fentanyl lolly for extreme burns where cannulation or oral morphine may be difficult should be debated. The military use this method but, again, it is an issue of the possession and supply that prevents paramedics from using this. With the lobbying that has recently encouraged the Home Office to look at ketamine there may be an opportunity to gather evidence nationwide about both of these issues and analyse the findings.

As a body representing and accountable to the public, the Ambulance Service and all staff representing the Ambulance Service have a role in ensuring pain is managed effectively, the importance of which cannot be understated.

Appendix 1

Current interventions

This guide has outlined a range of interventions that are accessible to practitioners working within the prehospital environment. Scopes of practice evolve over time and clinicians should work to the latest guidelines relevant for their particular role and under the guidance of the employer. When administering medication the latest indications, contraindications and cautions should be checked. New practice will inevitably be developed through research and innovation to ensure ongoing improvement in pain relief.

This table outlines some of the current interventions available.

	Intervention	Basic	Practitioner	Specialist	Advanced
Non-Pharmacological	Reassurance				
	Splinting				
	Positioning				
Pharmacological	Entonox				
	Paracetamol				
	Co-codamol				
	Codeine Phosphate				
	Dihydrocodeine				
	Morphine				
	Ketamine				
	Diclofenac				
	Ibuprofen				
	Lidocaine				
	Rizatriptan				
In-direct pain relieving effect	Aciclovir				
	Nystatin				
	Hyoscine Butylbromide				
	Glycerin Suppository				
	Lansoprazole				
	Ranitidine				
	Antacid				
	Alginate Reflux Suppressant				
	Diazepam				
	Midazolam				
	Prednisolone				

Appendix 2
Abbreviations

BASICS	British Association for Immediate Care Scheme
CCP	Specialist paramedic, critical care
CDs	Controlled drugs
CNS	Central nervous system
CPD	Continuous professional development
ECA	Emergency care assistant
ECP	Specialist paramedic, primary care
EMT	Emergency medical technician
GMC	General Medical Council
HEMS	Helicopter Emergency Medical Service
HPC	Health Professions Council
IHCD	Institute of Healthcare and Development
IM	Intramuscular
IV	Intravenous
JRCALC	Joint Royal Colleges Ambulance Liaison Committee
MHRA	Medicines and Healthcare Products Regulatory Agency
NSAID	Non-steroidal anti-inflammatory drug
QSAP	Qualified student ambulance paramedic
'RICE'	Rest, ice, compression, elevation
SAP	Student ambulance paramedic
SC	Subcutaneous
UN	United Nations

Bibliography

1. Shaw GB. The Doctor's Dilemma. 1906. In: Laurence D, ed. The Bodley Head Bernard Shaw: Collected Plays with Their Prefaces. Vol 3. London: Max Reinhardt, 1971:223–436.

2. http://www.nursingceu.com/courses/298/index_ot.html 15.8.11 Visited 12.8.11

3. Carr DB, Jacox AK, Chapman CR, Ferrell BR, Fields HL, Heidrich G III, Hester NK, Hill CS Jr., Lipman AG, McGarvey CL, Miaskowski CA, Mulder DS, Payne R, Schechter N, Shapiro BS, Smith RS, Tsou CV, Vecchiarelli L. Acute Pain Management: Operative or Medical Procedures and Trauma. Clinical Practice Guideline. Rockville, MD: Agency for Health Care Policy and Research, Public Health Service, US Department of Health and Human Services, 1992. AHCPR Pub. No. 92-0032.

4. Brennan F, et al: Pain Management: A Fundamental Human Right. A & A. Lippincot Williams and Wilkins. July 2007;105(1):205–221. Available at: http://www.anesthesiaanalgesia.org/content/105/1/205.full

5. MacIntyre P, on behalf of the Working Party of the Australian and New Zealand College of Anaesthetists. Acute Pain Management: Scientific Evidence, 2nd ed. Melbourne, Australia: Australian and New Zealand College of Anaesthetists, 2005. Available at: http://www.nhmrc.gov.au/publications/synopses/cp104syn.htm.

6. Descartes R. L'homme et un traitté de la formation du foetus du mesme autheur. Paris: C Angot; 1664.]

7. European Federation of IASP Chapters. EFIC's Declaration on Chronic Pain as a Major Healthcare Problem, a Disease in its Own Right. Presented at the European Parliament, Brussels, Belgium, October 9, 2001, after endorsement by 25 European Chapters of the International Society for the Study of Pain. Available at: http://www.painreliefhumanright.com/pdf/06_declaration.pdf.

8. Merskey H, Bogduk N. (Eds.) Classification of chronic pain: Description of chronic pain syndromes and definition of pain terms. Seattle: IASP Press, 1994.

9. Siddall PJ, Cousins MJ. Persistent pain as a disease entity: implications for clinical management. Anesth Analg 2004;99:510–20.

10. Gureje O, Von Korff M, Simon GE, Gater R. Persistent pain and well-being: a World Health Organization study in primary care. JAMA 1998;280:147–51.

11. Merskey H, Lau CL, Russell ES, Brooke RI, James M, Lappano S, Neilsen J, Tilsworth RH. Screening for psychiatric morbidity. The pattern of psychological illness and premorbid characteristics in four chronic pain populations. Pain 1987;30:141–57.

12. Fishbain D. Approaches to treatment decisions for psychiatric comorbidity in management of the chronic pain patient. Med Clin North Am 1999;83:737–60.

13. McMahon: Wall and Melzack's Textbook of Pain. Edinburgh: Churchill Livingstone; 5th revised edn, 2005.

14. McCaffrey M, Beebe A, Latham J (1994) Pain: A Clinical Manual for Nursing Practice. London: Mosby-Wolfe, 1994.

15. http://www.who.int/substance_abuse/research_tools/en/english_whoqol.pdf accessed 13.09.11

16. Seligman M.E.P. Helplessness: On Depression, Development, and Death. San Francisco: W.H. Freeman, 1975.

17. Thorpe DM. The incidence of sleep disturbance in cancer patients with pain. In: 7th World Congress on Pain: Abstracts. Seattle, WA: IASP Publications, 1993: abstract 451.

18. Cleeland CS, Nakamura Y, Mendoza TR, Edwards KR, Douglas J, Serlin RC. Dimensions of the impact of cancer pain in a four country sample: new information from multidimensional scaling. Pain 1996;67:267–73.

19. Feuz A, Rapin CH. An observational study of the role of pain control and food adaptation of elderly patients with terminal cancer. J Am Diet Assoc 1994;94:767–70.

20. Ferrell BR. The impact of pain on quality of life. A decade of research. Nurs Clin North Am 1995;30:609–24.

21. Katz N. The impact of pain management on quality of life. J Pain Symptom Manage 2002;24:S38.

22. Verhaak PF, Kerssens JJ, Dekker J, Sorbi MJ, Bensing JM. Prevalence of chronic benign pain disorder among adults: a review of the literature. Pain 1998;77:231–9.

23. Blyth FM, March LM, Brnabic AJM, Jorm LR, Williamson M, Cousins MJ. Chronic pain in Australia: a prevalence study. Pain 2001;89:127–34.

24. Stewart WF, Ricci JA, Chee E, Morganstein D, Lipton R. Lost productive time and cost due to common pain conditions in the US workforce. JAMA 2003;290:2443–54.

25. Van Leeuwen MT, Blyth FM, March LM, Nicholas MK, Cousins MJ. Chronic pain and reduced work effectiveness: the hidden cost to Australian employers. Eur J Pain 2006;2:161–6.

26. Blyth FM, March LM, Brnabic AJM, Cousins MJ. Chronic pain and frequent use of health care. Pain 2004;111:51–8.

27. Molloy AR, Blyth FM, Nicholas MK. Disability and work-related injury: time for a change? Med J Aust 1999;170:150–1.

28. Blyth FM, March LM, Nicholas MK, Cousins MJ. Chronic pain, work performance and litigation. Pain 2003;103:41–7.

29. Wittink H, Carr DB, eds. Pain Management: Evidence, Outcomes and Quality of Life. A Sourcebook. Amsterdam: Elsevier, 2005.

30. Ehrich EW, Bolognese JA, Watson DJ, Kong SX. Effect of rofecoxib on measures of shealth-related quality of life in patients with oasteoarthritis. Am J Manag Care 2001;7:609–16.

31. Rowbotham M, Harden N, Stacey B, Bernstein P, Magnus-Mille L. Gabapentin for the treatment of postherpetic neuralgia: a randomized controlled trial. JAMA 1998;280:1837–42.

32. Cousins MJ, Power I, Smith G. 1996 Labat Lecture: Pain—a persistent problem. Reg Anesth Pain Med 2000;25:6–21.

33. Dolin SJ, Cashman JN, Bland JM. Effectiveness of acute postoperative pain management. I. Evidence from published data. Br J Anaesth 2002;89:409–23.

34. Powell AE, Davies HT, Bannister J, Macrae WA. Rhetoric and reality on acute pain services in the UK: a national postal questionnaire survey. Br J Anaesth 2004;92:689–93.

35. The SUPPORT Principal Investigators. A controlled trial to improve care for seriously ill hospitalized patients. JAMA 1995;274:1591–8; erratum in JAMA 1996;275:1232.

36. Bardiau FM, Braeckman MM, Seidel L, Albert A, Boogaerts JG. Effectiveness of an acute pain service inception in a general hospital. J Clin Anesth 1999;11:583–9.

37. Gray PH, Trotter JA, Langbridge P, Doherty CV. Pain relief for neonates in Australian hospitals: a need to improve evidence-based practice. J Paediatr Child Health 2006;42:10–3.

38. Harrison D, Loughnan P, Johnston L. Pain assessment and procedural pain management practices in neonatal units in Australia. J Paediatr Child Health 2006;42:6–9.

39. Mather L, Mackie J. The incidence of postoperative pain in children. Pain 1983;15:271.

40. Crombie IK, Croft PR, Linton SJ, Le Resche L, Von Korff M, eds. Epidemiology of Pain. Seattle: IASP Press, 1999.

41. Won A, Lapane K, Gambassi G, Bernabei R, Mor V, Lipsitz LA. Correlates and management of non-malignant pain in the nursing home. J Am Geriatr Soc 1999;47:936–42.

42. Harstall C, Ospina M. How prevalent is chronic pain? Pain: Clin Updates 2003;11:1–4.

43. Sternbach RA. Survey of pain in the United States: the Nuprin Pain Report. Clin J Pain 1986;2:49–53.

44. Research!America. America Speaks: Pain in America. A survey among adults nationwide, August 2003. Available at: http://researchamerica.org/polldata/pain.html.

45. Teno JM, Weitzen S, Wetle T, Mor V. Persistent pain in nursing home residents [research letter]. JAMA 2001;285:208.

46. Selva C. International control of opioids for medical use. Eur J Palliat Care 1997;4:194–8.

47. Teoh N, Stjernsward J. WHO Cancer Pain Relief Program—Ten Years On. IASP Newsletter. Seattle: IASP Press, 1992; July/August: 5–6.

48. Goudas LC, Carr DB, Bloch R, Balk E, Ioannidis JPA, Terrin N, Gialeli-Goudas M, Chew P, Lau J. Management of Cancer Pain. Vols 1, 2. Evidence Tables. Evidence Report/Technology Assessment No. 35. Rockville, MD: Agency for Healthcare Research and Quality, 2001.

49. Daut RL, Cleeland CS. The prevalence and severity of pain in cancer. Cancer 1982;50:1913–8.

50. Ripamonti C, Dickerson ED. Strategies for the treatment of cancer pain in the new millennium. Drugs 2001;61:955–77.

51. Von Roenn JH, Cleeland CS, Gonin R, Hatfield AK, Pandya KJ. Physician attitudes and practice in cancer pain management: a survey from the Eastern Cooperative Oncology Group. Ann Intern Med 1993; 19:121–6.

52. Breitbart W, Rosenfeld BD, Passik SD, McDonald MV, Thaler H, Portenoy RK. The undertreatment of pain in ambulatory AIDS patients. Pain 1996; 65:243–9.

53. Carr DB, Goudas LC Evaluating and managing pain for patients with HIV/AIDS: an overview. In: Nedeljkovi SS, ed. Pain Management, Anesthesia, and HIV/AIDS. Boston: Butterworth-Heinemann, 2002:119–41, Chapter 10.

54. Carr DB. Fact Sheet on Pain in HIV/AIDS: A major global healthcare problem. European Federation of IASP Chapters 2004. Available at: http://www.efic.org/ 04B%20pain%20in%20HIV%20Fact%20Sheet.pdf.

55. Larue F, Colleau S, Brasseur L, Cleeland CS. Multicentre study of cancer pain and its treatment in France. BMJ 1995;310:1034–7.

56. Cleeland CS, Gonin R, Hatfield AK, Edmonson JH, Blum RH, Stewart JA, Pandya KJ. Pain and its treatment in outpatients with metastatic cancer. N Engl J Med 1994; 330:592–6.

57. Wang XS, Cleeland CS, Mendoza TR, Englstrom MC, Liu S, Xu G, Hao X, Wang Y, Ren XS. The effects of pain severity on health-related quality of life: a study of Chinese cancer patients. Cancer 1999; 86:1848–55.

58. Wolfe J, Grier HE, Klar N, Levin SB, Ellenbogen JM, Salem-Schatz S, Emanuel EJ, Weeks JC. Symptoms and suffering at the end of life in children with cancer. N Engl J Med 2000; 342:326–33.

59. Bonica JJ, Loeser JD. History of pain concepts and therapies. In: Loeser JD, Butler SH, Chapman CR, Turk DC, eds. Bonica's Management of Pain, 3rd edn. Philadelphia, PA: Lippincott, Williams and Wilkins, 2001:3–16.

60. Fulop-Miller R. Triumph over Pain. Translated by E and C Paul. London: Hamish Hamilton, 1938:7–8, 15–32.

61. Keele KD. Anatomies of Pain. Oxford: Blackwell 1957;1–16.

62. Procacci P, Maresca M. The pain concept in western civilization: a historical review. In: Benedetti C, Chapman CR, Moricca G, eds. Advances in the Management of Pain (Advances in Pain Research and Therapy. Vol 7). New York: Raven Press, 1984:17.

63. Rey R. History of Pain. Paris: Editions La Découverte, 1993.

64. Baszanger I. Inventing Pain Medicine: From the Laboratory to the Clinic. New Brunswick, NJ: Rutgers University Press, 1998.

65. Dormandy T. The Worst of Evils. New Haven: Yale University Press, 2006.

66. Carr DB. Letter to forum commenting on "Iceman from the Copper Age." Natl Geogr Mag 1993; 4:184.

67. Morris DB. The Culture of Pain. Berkeley, CA: University of California Press, 1994.

68. Papper EM. Romance, Poetry and Surgical Sleep: Literature Influences Medicine. Westport, CT: Greenwood Press, 1995.

69. Jacox AK, Carr DB, Payne R, Berde CB, Breitbart W, Cain JM, Chapman CR, Cleeland CS, Ferrell BR, Finley RS, et al. Management of Cancer Pain. Clinical Practice Guideline No. 9. Rockville, MD: Agency for Health Care Policy and Research, Public Health Service, US Department of Health and Human Services, 1994. AHCPR Pub. No. 94-0592.

70. Carr DB. The development of national guidelines for pain control: synopsis and commentary. Eur J Pain 2001; 5:91–8.

71. Warfield CA, Kahn CH. Acute pain management: programs in US hospitals and experiences and attitudes among US adults. Anesthesiology 1995; 83:1090–4.

72. Mitka M. "Virtual textbook" on pain developed: effort seeks to remedy gap in medical education. JAMA 2003; 290:2395.

73. European Federation of IASP Chapters. Unrelieved pain is a major global healthcare problem. 2004. Available at: http://www.efic.org/04A%20Global%20Day%20 Fact%20Sheet.pdf.

74. Melzack R IASP Presidential Address. The tragedy of needless pain: a call for social action. In: Dubner R, Gebbart MR, Bond MR, eds. Proceedings of the 5th World Congress of Pain. New York: Elsevier, 1988:1–11.

75. Body R, et al. The value of symptoms and signs in the emergent diagnosis of acute coronary syndromes. Resuscitation 2010;81(3),281–286.

76. International Narcotics Control Board. United Nations "Demographic Yearbook." Vienna: International Narcotics Control Board, 2005.

77. Pain and Policy Studies Group, WHO Collaborating Center for Policy and Communications in Cancer Care, University of Wisconsin Comprehensive Cancer Care Center. Opioid Analgesics—Trends, Guidelines, Resources. Prepared for the International Association for the Study of Pain, 10th World Congress on Pain, San Diego, CA, August 17–22, 2002. Available at: http://www.medsch.wisc.edu/ painpolicy/IASPmono.pdf.

78. James A. Painless human right. Lancet 1993;342:567–8.

79. Rich B. An ethical analysis of the barriers to effective pain management. Camb Q Healthc Ethics 2000;9:54.

80. Gilson AM, Joranson DE, Mauer MA. Improving medical board policies: influence of a model. J Law Med Ethics 2003;31:119–29.

81. Federation of State Medical Boards of the United States. Model policy for the Use of Controlled Substances for the Treatment of Pain. Dallas, TX; Federation of State Medical Boards of the United States, 2004. Available at: http://www.fsmb.org/ pdf/2004_grpol_Controlled_Substances.pdf.

82. de C Williams AC, Amris K, Van Der Merwe J. Pain in survivors of torture and organized violence. In: Dostrovsky JO, Carr DB, Koltzenburg M, eds. Proceedings of the 10th World Congress on Pain. Progress in Pain Research and Management. Vol 24. Seattle: IASP Press, 2003:791–802.

83. Lichtblau E. Justice Department opens inquiry into abuse of US detainees. New York Times, January 14, 2005, Late Edition, Section A, Column 3, National Desk, p 20.

84. Bennett D, Carr D. Opiophobia as a barrier to the treatment of pain. J Pain Palliat Care Pharmacother 2002; 16:105–9.

85. Ballantyne JC, Mao J. Opioid therapy for chronic pain. N Engl J Med 349; 20:1943–53.

86. McNicol E, Horowicz-Mehler N, Fisk RA, Bennett K, Gialeli-Goudas M, Chew PE, Lau J, Carr D. Management of opioid side effects in cancer-related and chronic noncancer pain—a systematic review. J Pain 2003; 4:231–56.

87. Pargeon KL, Hailey BJ. Barriers to effective cancer pain management: a review of the literature. J Pain Symptom Manage 1999; 18:358–68.

88. Martino AM. In search of a new ethic for treating patients with chronic pain: what can medical boards do? J Law Med Ethics 1998; 26:332–49.

89. Elliott TE, Elliott BA. Physician attitudes and beliefs about use of morphine for cancer pain. J Pain Symptom Manage 1992; 7:141–8.

90. Vainio A. Treatment of terminal care pain in France: a questionnaire study. Pain 1995; 62:155–62.

91. Ward SE, Goldberg N, Miller-McCauley V, Mueller C, Nolan A, Pawlik-Plank D, Robbins A, Stormoen D, Weissman DE. Patient related barriers to management of cancer pain. Pain 1993; 52:319–24.

92. Ward SE, Hernandez L. Patient-related barriers to cancer pain management in Puerto Rico. Pain 1994; 58:233–8.

93. Lin CC, Ward SE. Patient-related barriers to cancer pain management in Taiwan. Cancer Nurs 1995; 18:16–22.

94. Ziegler SJ, Lovrich NP Jr. Pain relief, prescription drugs, and prosecution: a four-state survey of chief prosecutors. J Law Med Ethics 2003; 31:75–100.

95. Carr DB, Loeser J, Morris DB, eds. Narrative, Pain and Suffering. Seattle: IASP Press, 2005.

96. Pernick MS. The calculus of suffering in nineteenth-century surgery. Hastings Cent Rep 1983; 13:26–36.

97. Council on Ethical and Judicial Affairs, American Medical Association. Decision near the end of life. JAMA 1992; 267:2229–33.

98. American Nurses Association. Code of Ethics for Nurses with Interpretive Statements. Washington, DC: American Nurses Publishing, 2001.

99. Post LF, Blustein J, Gordon E, Dubler NN. Pain: ethics, culture and informed consent to relief. J Law Med Ethics 1996; 24:348–59.

100. Somerville MA Death of pain: pain, suffering and ethics. In: Gebhart GF, Hammond DL, Jensen TS, eds. Proceedings of the 7th World Congress on Pain. Progress in Pain Research and Management. Vol 2. Seattle: IASP Press, 1994:41–58.

101. Cain JM, Hammes BJ. Ethics and pain management: respecting patient wishes. J Pain Symptom Manage 1994; 9:160–5.

102. Pecoul B, Chirac P, Trouiller P, Pinel J. Access to essential drugs in poor countries. A lost battle? JAMA 1999; 281:361–7.

103. Green CR, Anderson KO, Baker TA, Campbell LC, Decker S, Fillingim RB, Kaloukalani DA, Lasch KE, Myers C, Tait RC, Todd KH, Vallerand AH. The unequal burden of pain: confronting racial and ethnic disparities in pain. Pain Med 2003; 4:277–84.

104. Bentham J. In: Burns JH, Hart HLA (Eds). An Introduction to the Principles of Morals and Legislation. Oxford: Clarendon Press, 1996:343.

105. Weinman BP. Freedom from pain—establishing a constitutional right to pain relief. J Leg Med 2003; 24:495–539.

106. Medical Treatment Act 1994 (Australian Capital Territory), Section 23.

107. Consent to Medical Treatment and Palliative Care Act 1995 (South Australia), Sections 3 and 17(1).

108. Hyman CS. Pain management and disciplinary action: how medical boards can remove barriers to effective treatment. J Law Med Ethics 1996; 24:338–43.

109. California Business and Professional Code. s. 2190.5, 2241.6 and 2313. West, 2004.

110. Charatan F. New law requires doctors to learn care of the dying. BMJ 2001; 323:1088–9.

111. Assembly Bill 10407, 2003–2004 Session, New York, 2004.

112. The National Drug Authority (Prescription and Supply of Certain Narcotic Analgesic Drugs) Regulations, 2004. Statutory Instruments 2004, No. 24. Statutory Instruments Supplement to the Uganda Gazette No. 18. Vol XCVII.

113. Somerville MA. Death Talk. Montreal: McGill-Queen's University Press, 2001; 186:225–6.

114. Rich BA. Thinking the unthinkable: the clinician as perpetrator of elder abuse of patients in pain. J Pain Palliat Care Pharmacother 2004; 18:63–74.

115. California Welfare and Institute. Code. 15600–15675. West, 2004.

116. Dickens B. Commentary on 'Slow Euthanasia'. Journal of Palliative Care 1996; 12:43.

117. Von Gunten CF, Von Roenn JH. Barriers to pain control: ethics and knowledge. Journal of Palliative Care 1994; 10:52–4.

118. Somerville MA. Opioids for chronic pain of non-malignant origin—coercion or consent? Health Care Anal 1995; 3:12–14.

119. Emmanuel E. Pain and symptom control. Patient rights and physician responsibilities. Hematol Oncol Clin North Am 1996; 10:41–7.

120. Cousins MJ. Relief of acute pain: basic human right? Med J Aust 2000; 172:3.

121. Cousins MJ, Brennan F, Carr DB. Pain relief: a universal human right. Pain 2004; 112:1–4.

122. Alston P. The International Covenant on Economic, Social and Cultural Rights: Under Six Major International Human Rights Instruments. In: United Nations Centre For Human Rights and United Nations Institute for Training and Research. Manual on Human Rights Reporting. New York: United Nations, 1991:39.

123. Universal Declaration of Human Rights, 1948. United Nations General Assembly Resolution 217A (III). 1948.

124. Skene L. Law and Medical Practice—Rights, Duties, Claims and Defences. 2nd ed. Melbourne: Butterworths 2004; 56.

125. Queen's Bench Division, United Kingdom. Allinson v. General Council of Medical Education and Registration, 1894; 1:QB 750, 763.

126. New South Wales Court of Appeal. Pillai v. Messiter. 1989:16 NSWLR 197, at 202.

127. American Academy of Pain Medicine. Consent for Chronic Opioid Therapy. 1999. Available at: http://www.painmed.org/productpub/statements/pdfs/opioid_consent_form.pdf.

128. Berman S. (ed) Approaches to Pain Management: An Essential Guide for Clinical Leaders. Oakbrook Terrace, IL: Joint Commission on Accreditation of Healthcare Organizations, 2003.

129. Burgess FW. Pain scores: are the numbers adding up to quality patient care and improved pain control? Pain Med 2006; 7:371–2.

130. Vila H, Smith RA, Augustyniak MJ, Nagi PA, Soto RG, Ross TW, Cantor AB, Strickland JM, Miguel RV. The efficacy and safety of pain management before and after implementation of hospital-wide pain management standards: is patient safety compromised by treatment based solely on numerical pain ratings? Anesth Analg 2005; 101:474–80.

131. World Health Organization. Cancer Pain Relief. Geneva: WHO, 1986.

132. International Narcotics Control Board. Freedom from Pain and Suffering. Annual Report. Vienna: International Narcotics Control Board, 1999:2.

133. World Health Organization. National Cancer Control Programmes: Policies and Management Guidelines. 2nd ed. Geneva: WHO, 2002.

134. Dahl JL. Legal and regulatory aspects of opioid treatment: the United States experience. In: Brurera ED, Portenoy RK, eds. Cancer Pain. Assessment and Management. New York: Cambridge University Press, 2003; 458.

135. World Health Organization. Achieving balance in national opioids control policy— guidelines for assessment. Geneva: WHO, 2000.

136. Sepulveda C, Marlin A, Yoshida T, Ullrich A. Palliative care: the World Health Organization's perspective. J Pain Symptom Manage 2002; 24:91–6.

137. Dahl JL. Working with regulators to improve the standard of care in pain management: the US experience. J Pain Symptom Manage 2002; 24:136–47.

138. A Joint Statement from 21 Heath Organizations and the Drug Enforcement Administration. Promoting Pain Relief and Preventing Abuse of Pain Medication: A Critical Balancing Act. Available at: http://www.ampainsoc.org/advocacy/promoting. htm; http://www.ampainsoc.org/advocacy/pdf/consensus_1.pdf.

139. Dahl JL The state cancer pain initiative movement in the United States: successes and challenges. In: Meldrum M, ed. Opioids and Pain Relief: A Historical Perspective (Progress in Pain Research and Management. Vol 25). Seattle: IASP Press, 2003.

140. Stjernsward J, Clark D. Palliative medicine—a global perspective. In: Doyle D, Hanks G, Cherny N, Calman K, eds. Oxford Textbook of Palliative Medicine. 3rd Ed. New York: Oxford University Press, 2004:1199–222.

141. National Center for Health Statistics. Health, United States, 2006 With Chartbook on Trends in the Health of Americans. Hyattsville, MD: National Center for Health Statistics, 2006. Available at: http://www.cdc.gov/nchs/data/hus/hus06.pdf.

142. University of Sydney Graduate Studies Program in Pain Management. Available at: http://www.pmri.med.usyd.edu.au/education/degree_program.php.

143. Tufts University School of Medicine, Master of Science in Pain Research, Education and Policy. Available at: http://www.tufts.edu/med/education/phpd/msprep/index. html.

144. Ahmedzai SH, Costa A, Blengini C, Bosch A, Sanz-Ortiz J, Ventafridda V, Verhagen SC. A new international framework for palliative care. Eur J Cancer 2004; 40:2192–2200.

145. Montreal Statement on the Human Right to Essential Medicines. 2005. Available at: http://www.ccghr.ca/default.cfm?lang=e&content=accessmeds_news&subnav=news.

146. British House of Lords. Donoghue v Stevenson [1932]. 1932: AC 562.

147. Cousins MJ. Pain: The past, present, and future of anesthesiology? The E. A. Rovenstine Memorial Lecture. Anaesthesiology 1999; 91:538–51.

148. Linton SJ, McCracken LM, Vlaeyen JW. Reassurance: help or hinder in the treatment of pain. Pain. 2008; 134:5-8. Angst, MS & Clark, DJ: Opioid-induced hyperalgesia: A qualitative systematic review. Anesthesiology 2006; 104:570–87

149. Mao J: Opioid-induced abnormal pain sensitivity: Implications in clinical opioid therapy. Pain 2002; 100:213–7

150. Celerier E, Laulin J-P, Corcuff J-B, Le Moal M, Simonnet G: Progressive enhancement of delayed hyperalgesia induced by repeated heroin administration: A sensitization process. J Neurosci 2001; 21:4074–80

151. Chu LF, Angst MS, Clark D. Opioid-induced hyperalgesia in humans: molecular mechanisms and clinical considerations. Clin J Pain. 2008 Jul-Aug; 24(6):479-96. doi:10.1097/AJP.0b013e31816b2f43 PMID 18574358

152. Wuitchik, M. & Feehan, GG: Opioid withdrawal versus opioid maintenance for persons with chronic non-cancer pain: The experience of the Canmore Pain Clinic. Rehab Review 2006; 2:19-21

153. Drdla R, Gassner M, Gingl E, Sandkulher J. Induction Of Synaptic Long-Term Potentiation After Opiate Withdrawal. Science. 2009 Jul 10; 325(5937):207-10. doi:10.1126/science.1171759.

154. Amin A Algafly, Keith P George.The effect of cryotherapy on nerve conduction velocity, pain threshold and pain tolerance. British Journal of Sports Medicine 2007;41:365–369

155. Reid G, Babes A, Pluteanu F. A cold and menthol-activated current in rate dorsal root ganglion neurones: properties and role in cold transduction. J Physiol 2002; 545:595–614.

156. Carr ECJ, Mann E M (2000) Pain: Creative Approaches to Effective Management. Macmillan, Basingstoke.

157. Hawthorn J, Redmond K (1998) Pain: Causes and Management. Blackwell Science, Oxford

158. McCaffrey M, Beebe A, Latham J (1994) Pain: A Clinical Manual for Nursing Practice. Mosby-Wolfe, London.

159. National Council for Hospice and Specialist Palliative Care Services (2003) Priorities and Preferences for End of Life Care in England, Wales and Scotland. NCHSPCS, London

160. Jennings, PA, Cameron, P, Bernard, S. (2008), Measuring Acute Pain in the Prehospital Setting, Emergency Medical Journal, 2009:26, pp 552-555.

161. Lord, B and Woollard, M. (2010), The reliability of vital signs in estimating pain severity among adult patients treated by paramedics, Emergency medical Journal, [online], available from http://emj.bmj.com, [accessed 10th June 2011].

162. Royal College of Physicians, British Geriatrics Society and British Pain Society. The assessment of pain in older people: national guidelines. Concise guidance to good practice series, No 8. London: RCP, 2007.

163. Looker, J, Aldington D. (n.d.), Pain Scores – As easy as counting to Three, JR Army Med Corps, 155(1), pp42-67.

164. Fisher J D, Brown S N, Cooke M W. (2006), UK Ambulance Service Clinical Practice Guidelines, Joint Royal Colleges Ambulance Liaison Committee (JRCALC).

165. Herr, K. (2007), Pain Thermometer Scale Overview, Professional Postgraduate Services, [online], available from http://www.painknowledge.org, [accessed 4th September 2011].

166. The National Initiative on Pain Control, (n.d.), Pain Assessment Scales, Thompson Professional Postgraduate Services

167. Feldt, KS. (2000), The checklist of nonverbal pain indicators (CNPI). Pain Management Nursing, 1(1): 13-21.

168. Fuchs-Lacelle, S and Hadjistavropoulos, T (2007), PASLAC

169. McGrath, PJ and Johnson, G. (1985), A behavioural scale of rating postoperative pain in Children, Adv Pain Research Therapy, 1985:9, pp395-402.

170. Beyer, J. (1983), OUCHER, [online], available from http://www.oucher.org, [accessed 4th September 2011].

171. Warden, V Hurley, AC, Volicer, L. (2003), Development and Psycometric evaluation of the pain assessment in advanced dementia (PAINAD) scale. J M Med Dir Assoc., 2003:4, pp9-15

172. Melzack, R. (1970), McGill Pain Questionnaire: Major properties and scoring methods. Pain, 1975; 1, pp 277-299.

173. Charles, S Cleeland PD. (1991), British Pain Inventory (short form), Pain Research Group: Department of Neuro-Oncology, The University of Texas MD Anderson Cancer Centre

174. British Pain Society and British Geriatrics Society. Guidance on: The assessment of pain in older people. London: BPS/BGS, 2007.

175. Association of Paediatric Anaesthetists of Great Britain and Ireland, The British Pain Society, Royal College of Paediatrics and Child Health. The recognition and assessment of acute pain in children: Update of full guideline, Improving Practice: Improving Care-Clinical Practice Guidelines, London: Royal College of Nursing, 2009.

176. Faces Pain Scale (Bieri D, Reeve RA, Champion GD, Addicoat L, Ziegler JB. The Faces Pain Scale for the self-assessment of the severity of pain experienced children: Development, initial validation, and preliminary investigation for ratio scale properties. Pain, 1990;41:139–150.

177. Advanced Life Support Group (Mackway-Jones K, Molyneux E, Phillips B, Weiteska S. (2008), Advanced Paediatric Life Support: The practical Approach, 4th edn. Oxford: Blackwell Publishing, 2008.

178. Neuroscience online. http://neuroscience.uth.tmc.edu/s2/chapter06.html accessed 1.11.11

179. Buskila D, Sarzi-Puttini P, Ablin JN. 2007. The genetics of fibromyalgia syndrome: Pharmacogenomics, 2007;8(1):67–74.

180. Department of Health National Service Framework for Children Young People and Maternity Services: Children and Young People; section 6, 2007 http://www.dh.gov.uk/en/Publicationsandstatistics/Publications/PublicationsPolicyAn dGuidance/Browsable/DH_4867919 accessed 1.11.11

181. UK Ambulance Service Clinical Practice Guidelines. Joint Royal Colleges Ambulance Liaison Committee (JRCALC). October 2006

182. http://www.mhra.gov.uk (accessed 1.11.11)

183. Milne RW, Nation RL, Somogyi AA, Bochner F, Griggs WM. The influence of renal function on the renal clearance of morphine and its glucuronide metabolites in intensive-care patients. Br. J. clin. Pharmac, 1992;34:53–59

184. http://www.dailymail.co.uk/health/article-1153356/How-lollipop-helping-Jade-beat-pain-cancer.html (accessed 1.11.11)

185. Campagna JA, Miller KW, Forman SA. Mechanisms of actions of inhaled anasthetics. N Engl J Med, 2003; 348:2110–2124.

186. Melzack R, Wall PD. Pain mechanisms: a new theory. Science, 1965;150(3699):971–9.

187. Gibson SJ, Helme RD. Age-related differences in pain perception and report. Clin Geriatr Med 2001; 17:433–456.

188. Post LF, Blustein J, Gordon E, Dubler NN. Pain: ethics, culture and informed consent to relief. J Law Med Ethics 1996;24:348–59.

189. Skills for Health. Competence and Curriculum Framework for the Emergency Care Practitioner. Bristol: ECP Team, Skills for Health, 2007.

190. Tyring SK, Beutner KR, Tucker BA, et al. Antiviral therapy for herpes zoster: randomized, controlled clinical trial of valacyclovir and famciclovir therapy in immunocompetent patients 50 years and older. Arch Fam Med, 2000; 9(9):863–9.

191. Anthony T, Baron T, Mercadante S, et al. Report of the clinical protocol committee: development of randomized trials for malignant bowel obstruction. J Pain Symptom Manage, 2007; 34(1 Suppl): S49–59.

192. Ripamonti CI, Easson AM, Gerdes H. Management of malignant bowel obstruction. Eur J Cancer, 2008; 44(8):1105–15.

193. Jimenez N, Bradford H, Seidel KD, et al. A comparison of a needle-free injection system for local anesthesia versus EMLA for intravenous catheter insertion in the pediatric patient. Anesth Analg, 2006; 102(2):411–4.

194. Lysakowski C, Dumon TL, Tramèr MR, Tassonyi E, et al. A needle-free jet-injection system with lidocaine for peripheral intravenous cannula insertion: a randomized controlled trial with cost-effectiveness analysis. Anesth Analg, 2003; 96(1):215–9.

195. Hogan ME, vanderVaart S, Perampaladas K. Systematic review and meta-analysis of the effect of warming local anesthetics on injection pain. Ann Emerg Med, 2011; 58(1):86–98.

196. Oldman AD, Smith LA, McQuay HJ, et al. Pharmacological treatments for acute migraine: quantitative systematic review. Pain, 2002; 97(3):247–57.

197. Targownik. L.E., Metge. C.J., Leung. S. et al The relative efficacies of gastroprotective strategies in chronic users of nonsteroidal anti-inflammatory drugs. Gastroenterology, 2008;134(4):937–44.

198. Harris T, Cameron PA, Ugoni A. The use of pre-cannulation anaesthetic and factors affecting pain perception in the emergency department setting. Emerg Med, 2001;18: 175–7.

199. Robinson PA, Carr S, Pearson S, Frampton C. Lignocaine is a better analgesic than either ethyl chloride or nitrous oxide for peripheral intravenous cannulation. Emergency Medicine Australasia, 2007;19:427–432.

200. National Health And Medical Research Council & Australian Acute Musculoskeletal Pain Guidelines Group. Evidence-based Management of Acute Musculoskeletal Pain. Brisbane: Australian Academic Press, 2003.

201. Romsing J, Moiniche S, Dahl JB. Rectal and parenteral paracetamol, and paracetamol incombination with NSAIDs, for postoperative analgesia. Br J Anaesth, 2002; 88(2):215–26.

202. Marjoribanks J, Proctor ML., Farquhar C. Nonsteroidal anti-inflammatory drugs for primary dysmenorrhoea. Cochrane Database Syst Rev, 2003;4: CD001751.

203. Hyllested M, Jones S, Pedersen JL, et al. Comparative effect of paracetamol, NSAIDs or their combination in postoperative pain management: a qualitative review. Br J Anaesth, 2002;88(2):199–214.

204. Kumar A, Deed JS, Bhasin B, et al. Comparison of the effect of diclofenac with hyoscine-Nbutylbromide in the symptomatic treatment of acute biliary colic. ANZ J Surg, 2004; 74(7):573–6.

205. Holdgate A, Pollock T. Nonsteroidal anti-inflammatory drugs (NSAIDs) versus opioids for acute renal colic. Cochrane Database Syst Rev, 2005;2: CD004137.

206. Whitley RJ, Weiss H, Gnann JW, et al. Acyclovir with and without prednisone for the treatment of herpes zoster. A randomized, placebo-controlled trial. The National Institute of Allergy and Infectious Diseases Collaborative Antiviral Study Group. Ann Intern Med, 1996; 125(5):376–83.

207. Benedetti F, Arduino C, Amanzio M. Somatotopic activation of opioid systems by target-directed expectations of analgesia. J Neuroscience, 1999; 19:3639–48.

208. Horgas AL,Tsai PF. Analgesic drug prescription and use in cognitively impaired nursing home residents. Nursing Research, 1998; 47: 235–242.

209. Carr ECJ, Mann EM. Pain: Creative Approaches to Effective Management. Basingstoke: Macmillan, 2000.

Index